THE AMERICAN BLUE ZONE COOKBOOK

A Complete Longevity Diet Guide with Healthy Delicious Recipes, Food Lists, and a 28-day Meal Plan for Beginners, to Live to 100 and Beyond.

Also by Dr. Angela Cook

Scan the QR code to see other books by Dr. Angela Cook.

THE AMERICAN BLUE ZONES COOKBOOK

A Complete Longevity Diet Guide with Healthy Delicious Recipes, Food Lists, and a 28-day Meal Plan for Beginners, to Live to 100 and beyond.

DR. ANGELA COOK

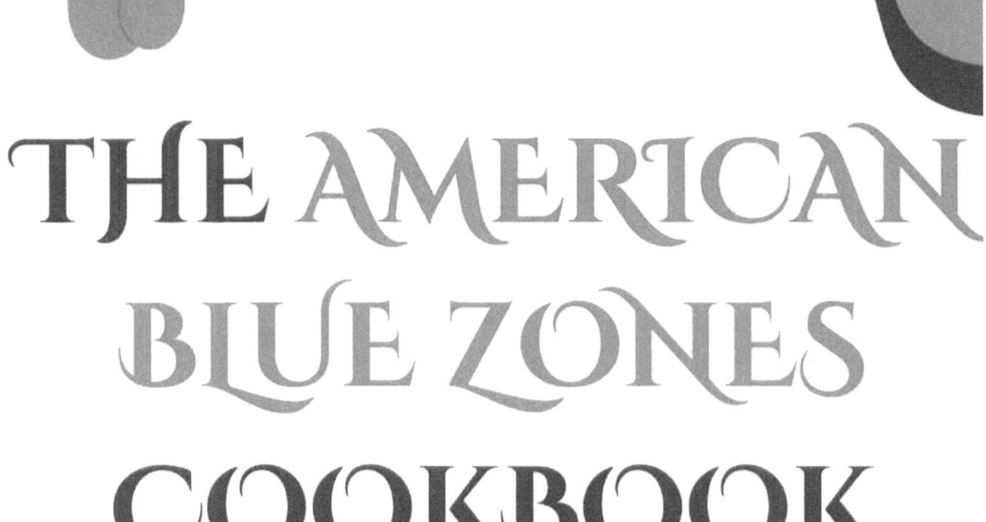

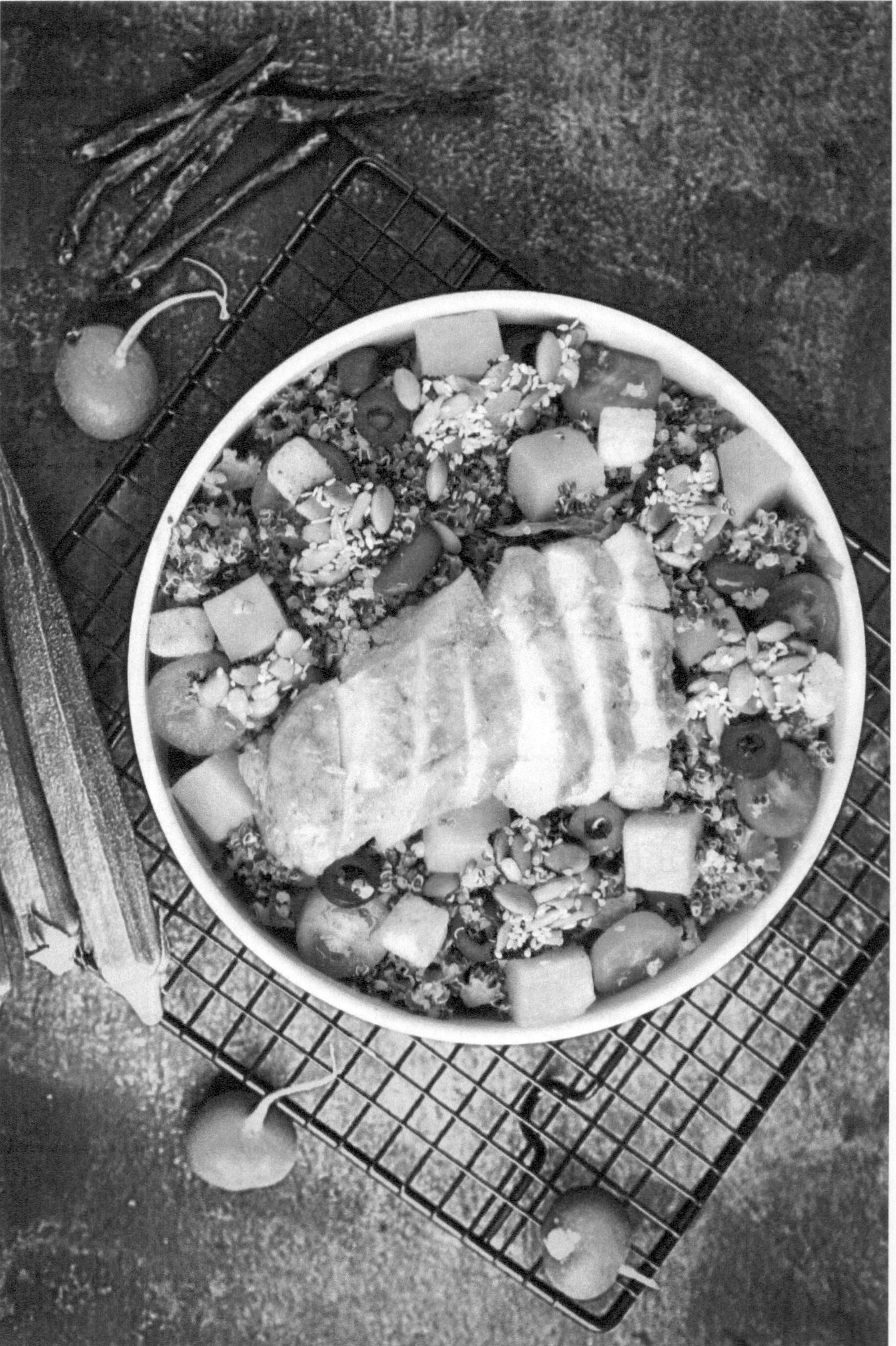

The recipes in this cookbook are provided as a guide for those interested in the Mediterranean diet. Individual dietary needs and preferences may vary, and it is important to adapt these recipes to your specific requirements.

The author and publisher do not endorse any specific products, brands, or services mentioned in this cookbook, and any product recommendations are for informational purposes only.

The information provided in this cookbook is for general informational and educational purposes only. While every effort has been made to ensure the accuracy and completeness of the content, the author and publisher make no representations or warranties of any kind, express or implied, about the suitability, applicability, or reliability of the recipes, nutritional information, tips, or guidelines presented.

Dedication

To all those on the quest for a life well-lived, marked by vitality, joy, and the simple pleasures of nourishing the body and soul, this dedication page stands as a testament to your commitment.

In homage to the resilient spirit within each of us, may this collection of Blue Zones-inspired recipes be a guide on your journey to longevity and well-being. Dedicated to the seekers of balance and the embracers of cultural wisdom, may every dish on these pages reflect the essence of a life filled with health and connection.

This work is dedicated to the explorers of flavor, the stewards of their own well-being, and to those who find joy in the art of crafting a meal that not only sustains but also enriches life's tapestry.

May you continue to savor each moment and every bite, with the dedication to a life abundant in good health, shared meals, and the profound wisdom of the Blue Zones. Here's to your journey of dedication and the celebration of a life well-nourished.

With heartfelt dedication,

Dr. Angela Cook

How to Use This Book

1. **Explore and Absorb:** Begin your journey by immersing yourself in the introductory chapters. Dive into the evolution of the American diet and grasp the essence of the Blue Zones philosophy. Understand the guidelines and advantages offered by this transformative approach to eating.

2. **Plan and Prep:** Engage with the comprehensive 28-Day Meal Plan meticulously designed for your convenience. Use it as a blueprint to structure your weeks, ensuring a seamless integration of nutritious meals into your routine.

3. **Navigate the Recipes:** Discover a treasure trove of recipes divided into breakfasts, soups, salads, main courses, and desserts. Feel free to navigate according to your preferences or dietary needs.

4. **Choose Your Adventure:** Select recipes that pique your interest or align with your cravings. Dive into the flavors of the Blue Zones with diverse dishes, each crafted to bring a taste of longevity and vitality to your table.

5. **Embrace Variety:** Embrace the variety offered within these pages. Experiment with different cuisines, ingredients, and cooking styles. Let each recipe be an exploration of flavor and a celebration of nourishment.

6. **Personalize and Enjoy:** Make each recipe your own. Personalize them by adding a personal twist or adapting them to suit your taste preferences. Most importantly, savor every bite and relish the joy that comes with preparing and enjoying wholesome meals.

7. **Share the Experience:** Share this culinary adventure with loved ones. Invite friends and family to join you on this journey towards a healthier, more vibrant lifestyle. Food, after all, is best enjoyed when shared.

8. **Refer and Repeat:** Keep this book handy as a go-to resource in your kitchen. Refer back to it whenever you seek inspiration or wish to revisit your favorite recipes. Repeat the recipes that resonate most with you and integrate them into your regular meal rotations.

9. **Celebrate Progress:** Celebrate each step you take towards a healthier lifestyle. Notice the changes in how you feel, both physically and mentally, as you nourish your body with the wisdom of the Blue Zones.

10. **Continue the Journey:** Remember, this book is not just a collection of recipes—it's a guide to a lifelong journey of wellness. Let it be a companion as you continue to prioritize your health, embrace the joy of cooking, and savor the abundance of a life well-lived.

11. **Write a Review:** You don't have to wait till after experiencing the transformative power of these recipes before you share your thoughts and experiences by writing a review. Your feedback can inspire others to embark on their own culinary journey towards wellness. Let your review be a testament to the flavors, nourishment, and joy this book has brought into your life. Your words might encourage someone else to take their first steps towards a healthier, more vibrant lifestyle.

Contents

INTRODUCTION

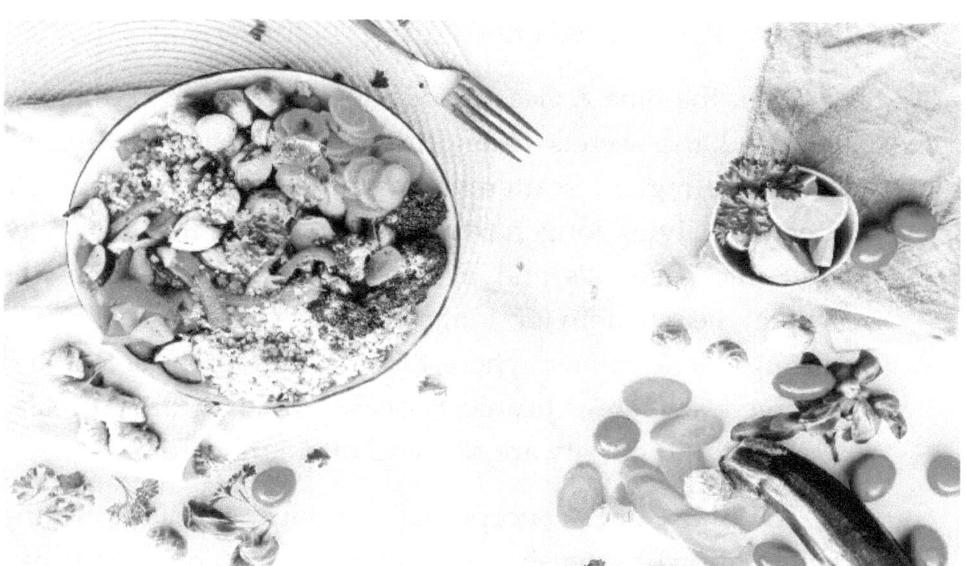

This book could help you unlock the secret to living an extra 10 good years. In 2022, the unfortunate reality is that a staggering 750,000 Americans will meet their untimely demise due to the consequences of consuming a standard American diet. Among these tragic losses, nearly 48,000 souls will succumb to the silent killer known as high blood pressure, and an alarming 213,000 lives will be cut short by the insidious grip of obesity. The statistics are staggering, and the toll on human lives and well-being is immeasurable.

But what would it feel like if there were a way to reform this narrative? What if we could learn from those among us who have cracked the code to living long, healthy lives?

What if the key to longevity isn't hidden in some distant, unattainable realm but is instead rooted in our everyday choices, particularly in the food we put on our plates and share with our loved ones?

Enter the Blue Zones, a groundbreaking concept that has unveiled the secrets to enduring vitality and well-being. These are regions scattered across the globe where people aren't just living longer; they're living better, healthier lives well into their 90s and even 100s. These are the places where the wisdom of longevity has been passed down through generations, where the elderly remain active and engaged, where chronic diseases like heart disease, diabetes, and obesity are rare and often unheard of.

The Blue Zones concept was not born overnight; it's the culmination of extensive research conducted by experts like Dan Buettner, and his dedicated team. They embarked on a journey to uncover the lifestyle and dietary habits of these remarkable communities.

I and my team were overwhelmed by this amazing discovery. So, our quest took us to Okinawa, Japan, where the island's centenarians offered insights into their plant-based diet, rich in vegetables and nutrient-dense foods. We ventured to Sardinia, Italy, a Mediterranean haven where the inhabitants thrive on whole grains, healthy fats, and a vibrant sense of community. In Loma Linda, California, we met the Adventists, who've harnessed the power of a plant-centric diet to maintain their vitality. Nicoya, Costa Rica, revealed its secrets, showing us how simple, unprocessed ingredients can make a world of difference in one's health. And on the Greek island of Ikaria, we discovered the Mediterranean way of living, replete with fresh vegetables, olive oil, and a slower, more mindful pace.

Now, you might wonder how these far-flung locales connect to the way your grandparents and great-grandparents lived in America. The answer lies in the remarkable similarities between the dietary and lifestyle choices made by the Blue Zones residents and those who lived in the United States before the era of fast food, processed snacks, and sedentary living.

Think back to the stories your grandparents or great-grandparents shared with you about their lives. Chances are, they grew their own vegetables, savored home-cooked meals, and engaged in physical labor or daily walks to get around. Their meals were hearty, filled with whole grains, fresh fruits and vegetables, and lean proteins. They embraced the joy of community gatherings and cherished the bonds of family. The difference between their way of life and the fast-paced, convenience-oriented culture we find ourselves in today is profound.

As I embarked on this journey of discovery, I couldn't help but draw parallels between the traditional American way of life, as remembered by our forebears, and the lifestyles I witnessed in the Blue Zones. There's a remarkable symmetry in the values of our ancestors and those living in these pockets of longevity. It's a testament to the enduring wisdom of generations past, and a testament to the fact that the keys to a long, fulfilling life are often hidden in plain sight.

This book, "The American Blue Zones Cookbook: 100 Recipes to Live to 100," is our attempt to bridge this connection, to rekindle the traditions of wholesome, nourishing eating that once defined American households. We aim to take the principles of the Blue Zones and bring them to your table, showing you that the path to a longer, healthier life is not an arduous one. In fact, it's as simple as preparing and sharing meals that honor the time-tested wisdom of our ancestors and the time-honored traditions of Blue Zones communities.

The significance of diet in promoting longevity and well-being cannot be overstated. What you put on your plate today can impact not only how long you live but how well you live. It can influence your vitality, your energy levels, your ability to ward off disease, and your overall sense of happiness. In this book, we're not just offering you a collection of recipes; we're offering you a journey toward a better, more fulfilling life.

In the pages that follow, you'll find a treasure trove of recipes inspired by the Blue Zones, categorized by meal type: breakfasts, soups and stews, salads and sides, main courses, and desserts. Each recipe is a testament to the culinary heritage of the world's longest-living populations, and each one is designed to help you incorporate their time-tested wisdom into your daily life. With these recipes, you can make the choice to nourish your body, elevate your well-being, and extend your health span.

But this book is not just about recipes. It's about a way of life, a way of eating that transcends the limitations of fad diets and quick fixes. It's about embracing the enduring wisdom of the Blue Zones and your own heritage. It's about creating a Blue Zones-inspired kitchen that becomes the heart of your home, a place where you gather with family and friends, share stories, and savor delicious, healthful meals.

So, are you ready to embark on a journey toward living a longer, healthier, and more fulfilling life? Are you ready to experience the magic of the Blue Zones right in your own home? If so, turn the page and let's begin this transformative adventure together. The power to change your life for the better is in your hands, and it all starts with what you choose to put on your plate.

EVOLUTION OF THE AMERICAN DIET

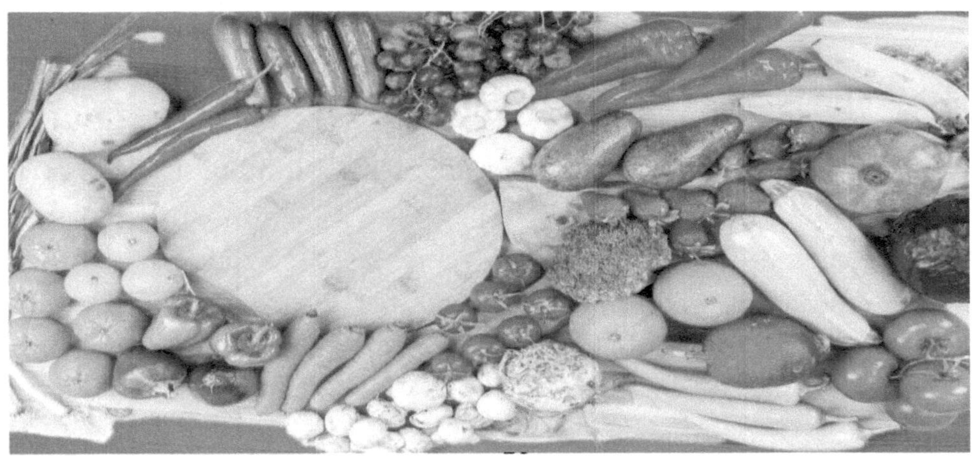

The history of how the American diet has evolved from the way Native Americans used to eat in the past is a complex narrative that spans centuries. It's a tale of profound transformation, driven by the collision of cultures, the influx of new ingredients, and the rise of industrialization. To comprehend this shift, we need to delve into the following key phases:

1. Pre-European Contact: Traditional Native American Diets

Prior to the arrival of European settlers, Native Americans inhabited a diverse range of ecosystems across North America. Their diets were strongly influenced by their environment, with each region offering a unique bounty of foods. Native Americans were skilled hunters, gatherers, and farmers, and they had a deep understanding of sustainable agriculture and resource management. Common dietary staples included maize (corn), beans, and squash, known as the "Three Sisters," along with wild game, fish, fruits, and vegetables. Native American diets were characterized by their reliance on unprocessed, whole foods, and a balanced mix of macronutrients.

2. The Columbian Exchange: Introduction of New Ingredients

With the arrival of Christopher Columbus in 1492 and subsequent European explorers, the Columbian Exchange began. This marked the interchange of foods and other goods between the Old World and the New World. While it led to the global spread of various crops and livestock, it also had a profound impact on Native American diets. New World foods like maize, potatoes, tomatoes, and peppers were introduced to Europe, while Old World items such as wheat, sugar, and livestock arrived in the Americas. This exchange of crops had lasting consequences for the dietary landscape in both regions.

3. Colonial Period: Shift Toward European-Influenced Diets

As European settlers established colonies across North America, they brought their own culinary traditions and agricultural practices. The cultivation of wheat, along with the introduction of dairy and various livestock, began to reshape the diet of the Native American populations. Native Americans adapted to these new foods, but it marked a significant departure from their traditional diets. The shift towards a more European-influenced diet included an increased consumption of refined grains, meat, and dairy products.

4. Westward Expansion and Frontier Life: Simplified and Preserved Foods

During the westward expansion of the United States, settlers faced the challenges of frontier life. The need for foods that could be easily preserved and transported led to the increased consumption of processed and canned foods. Traditional Native American dietary practices, which emphasized fresh, locally sourced ingredients, were often compromised in the face of these new dietary norms.

5. Industrialization and Convenience Foods: Mass Production and Processing

The late 19th and early 20th centuries saw the rapid industrialization of food production. This era brought about the mass production of processed foods, such as canned goods, white bread, and sugar-laden products. Convenience became a driving force in the American diet, leading to a reliance on foods high in sugar, salt, and unhealthy fats. As a result, diets became increasingly devoid of essential nutrients and laden with empty calories.

6. Post-World War II: Rise of Fast Food and Convenience Culture

The post-World War II period witnessed the proliferation of fast-food chains and the emergence of a convenience culture. Fast food, with its high-fat, high-sugar, and high-salt offerings, became a dominant feature of American eating habits. Portion sizes expanded, and the consumption of sugary beverages surged, contributing to the growing prevalence of obesity and diet-related diseases.

7. Modern Dietary Challenges: The Standard American Diet (SAD)

Today, the American diet is often characterized by the Standard American Diet (SAD). It is heavy in processed foods, red and processed meats, refined grains, sugar-sweetened beverages, and unhealthy fats. This diet has been linked to a rising epidemic of diet-related health issues, including obesity, heart disease, type 2 diabetes, and certain cancers. Native American populations, who were originally stewards of balanced, whole-food diets, have

CHAPTER 1: DIET GUIDE

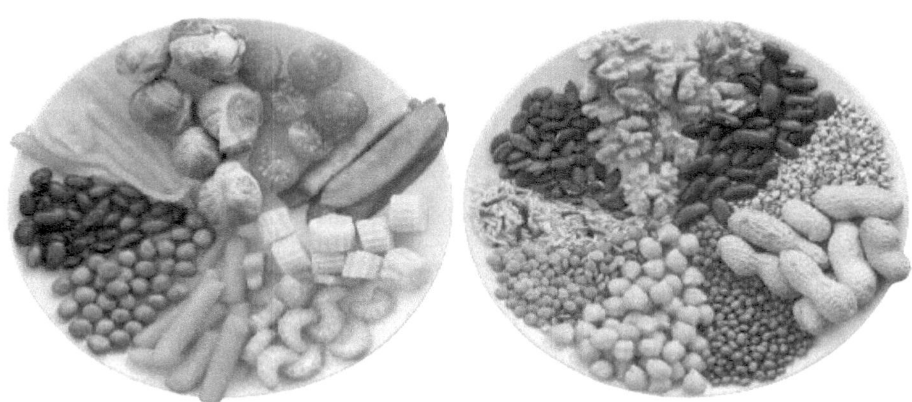

There are five blue zones on the planet where people enjoy long and healthy lives. They all have some common lifestyle habits, but they are all unique.

Greece, Ikaria: Ikaria is an island in the Eastern Aegean Sea notable for its high number of centenarians. Ikarians have low chronic disease rates and eat a diet high in vegetables, lentils, olive oil, and herbal teas.

Japan's Okinawa: Okinawa, a Japanese island chain, is known for its long life expectancy and large number of centenarians. Okinawan cuisine features a wide range of vegetables, tofu, sweet potatoes, and shellfish. Their lifespan is partly ascribed to the cultural practice of "Hara Hachi Bu," which encourages ending eating when 80% full.

Italy's Sardinia: Sardinia's hilly terrain, especially the Barbagia region, has a significant proportion of centenarians. Whole grains, legumes, veggies, and goat's milk are staples of the traditional Sardinian diet. Their well-being is enhanced by regular physical activity and strong community relationships.

Costa Rica's Nicoya Peninsula: Costa Rica's Nicoya Peninsula boasts a higher-than-average life expectancy. The Nicoyan diet consists primarily of beans, corn, and squash. Regular physical exercise, deep social relationships, and a sense of purpose characterize their way of life.

Loma Linda, California, United States: Loma Linda is a Southern California neighborhood notable for its Seventh-day Adventist population, which has a higher life expectancy than the average American population. The Adventist diet focuses on plant-based meals, nuts, and healthy living habits.

1. Beans on a daily basis

Consume a minimum of 1/2 cup of prepared beans every day.

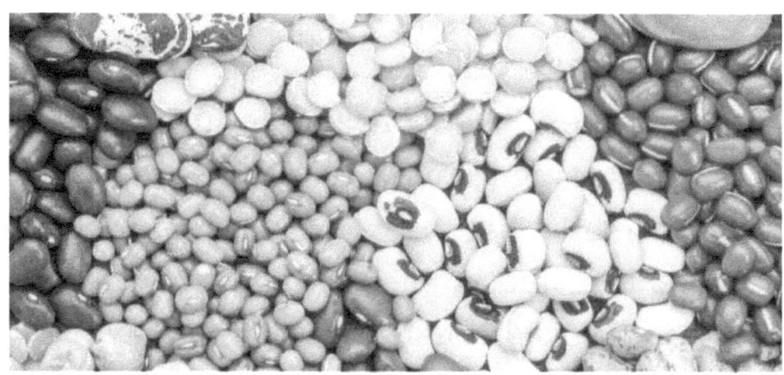

Black beans in Nicoya Island; lentils, garbanzo, and white beans in the Mediterranean; and soybeans in Okinawa constitute the foundation of every Blue Zones diet around the world. Lasting populations in these blue zones consume at least four times as much beans as we do. One World Health Organization-funded five-country study discovered that eating 20 grams of beans daily lowered a person's risk of dying by around 8% in any given year.

Ways you can accomplish it:

- As part of a Blue Zones diet, find ways to cook beans that taste delicious to you and your family. Blue zone centenarians know how to make beans taste wonderful. If you don't already have your favorite bean dishes, make a resolution to try three new ones in the next month.

- Stock your kitchen cupboard with a range of ready-to-eat beans. Dry beans are the cheapest, but canned beans cook faster. When purchasing canned beans, always read the label: Beans, water, spices, and sometimes a little salt should be the only components. Avoid brands that have additional fat or sugar.
- On the Blue Zones diet, use pureed beans as a thickening to make dishes creamy and protein-rich.
- To make salads more full, add cooked beans. To add texture and appeal to salads, serve hummus or black bean cakes alongside.
- Keep condiments in your cabinet to spice up bean recipes and make them taste fantastic. Mediterranean bean dishes, for example, typically include carrots, celery, and onion that have been seasoned with garlic, thyme, pepper, and bay leaves. This is a simple method to add variety to a Blue Zones diet.
- When dining out, look for Mexican eateries, which nearly always feature pinto or black beans. Add rice, onions, peppers, guacamole, and hot sauce to the beans to make them more flavorful. White flour tortillas should be avoided. Instead, choose maize tortillas, which are used to eat beans in Costa Rica.

2. Reduce Sugar

Consume no more than seven tablespoons of additional sugar each day.

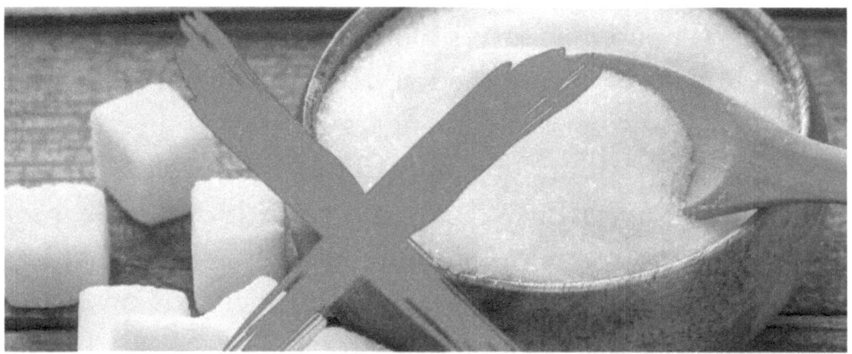

Centenarians often consume sweets only on special occasions. Their dishes are sugar-free, and they usually sweeten their tea using honey. Regarding the Blue Zones diet, this amounts to around seven teaspoons of sugar per day. The moral of the story: Cookies, sweets, and bakery items should be consumed only a few times each week, ideally as part of a meal. Sugary foods should be avoided. Any product with sugar as one of the first five components should be avoided. Sugar used in coffee, tea, or other types of beverages should not exceed four tablespoons per day. Get out of the habit of munching on sugary treats.

Ways you can accomplish it:

- Honey should be your go-to sweetener for the Blue Zones diet. Although honey raises blood sugar levels in the same way that sugar does, it is more difficult to incorporate and does not dissolve as well in cold liquids. As a result, you tend to consume food more deliberately and consume less of it. Honey is a whole food with anti-inflammatory, anticancer, and antibacterial effects, such as Ikarian heather honey.

- Avoid sugary sodas, teas, and fruit drinks entirely. Sugar-sweetened soda is the single most abundant source of added sugars in our diet; in fact, soft drink consumption may be responsible for half of America's weight gain since 1970. One can of soda pop contains around ten tablespoons of sugar. If you must consume soda, go for diet soda or, even better, seltzer or sparkling water.
- As a celebration snack, eat sweets. People in blue zones enjoy sweets, although sweets (cookies, cakes, pies, and various desserts) are nearly always served as a celebration food—after a Sunday meal, as part of a religious holiday, or at village festivals. In fact, special sweets are frequently available on these occasions. Desserts or pastries should be no more than 100 calories. Consume a maximum of one portion per day.
- Think of fruit as your sweet treat when following a Blue Zones diet at home. Fresh fruit is preferable to dried fruit. Fresh fruit contains more water and makes you feel fuller while consuming fewer calories. Sugars are concentrated far beyond what you would get in a typical serving of fresh fruit in dried fruit, such as raisins and dates.

- Be wary of sugary processed foods, particularly sauces, salad dressings, and ketchup. Many have several tablespoons of sugar added.
- Be wary of low-fat items, as many of them are sugar-sweetened to compensate for the loss of fat. Some low-fat yogurts, for example, have more sugar per ounce than soda pop.
- If you can't get your sweet tooth to go away, try stevia to sweeten your tea or coffee. Of course, it's not an actual Blue Zones diet, but it's very concentrated, so it's definitely better than refined sugar.

3. Plant Based

Make sure that 95% of your diet is derived from a plant or a plant product.

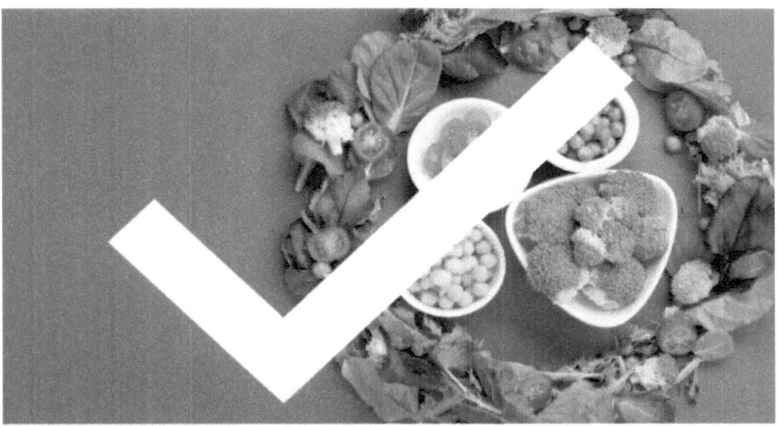

Limit your intake of animal protein to one tiny dish per day. Beans, greens, yams, sweet potatoes, fruits, nuts, and seeds are all good choices. Whole grains are also OK. People in four of the five blue zones eat meat, but only in moderation, as a festive food, a tiny side dish, or to flavor foods.

Indeed, studies show that 30-year-old vegetarian Adventists survive their meat-eating counterparts by up to eight years. Simultaneously, increasing the amount of plant-based foods in your diet provides numerous health benefits. People in the blue zones eat a wide variety of garden vegetables when they are in season, and then pickle or dry the excess to enjoy during the off-season. Leafy greens such as spinach, kale, beet and turnip tops, chard, and collards are among the finest lifespan foods in the Blue Zones diet. More than 75 species of edible greens grow like weeds on Ikaria, with many containing ten times the polyphenols found in red wine. According to studies, middle-aged adults who ate the equivalent of a cup of cooked greens daily were half as likely to die in the next four years as those who did not eat any greens.

Researchers also discovered that persons who ate a quarter pound of fruit each day (about an apple) were 60% less likely to die over the next four years than those who did not.

Many oils are derived from plants, and they are all preferable to fats derived from animals. Although we cannot claim that olive oil is the only healthy plant-based oil, it is the most commonly used in the Blue Zones diet.

Olive oil usage appears to raise good cholesterol while decreasing bad cholesterol.

Ways you can accomplish it:

- Fill up your home with your preferred fruits and vegetables. Try not to force yourself to consume foods you dislike. That may work for a while, but it will eventually fail. Try a variety of fruits and vegetables; learn the ones you prefer and keep them in your kitchen. If you don't have access to fresh, inexpensive vegetables, frozen vegetables will suffice.
- Treat olive oil like you would butter. Use olive oil to Sauté the vegetables over low flame. Finish steamed or boiled veggies by drizzling them with extra-virgin olive oil, which you should keep on hand.
- Increase your intake of whole grains. We discovered that oats, barley, brown rice, and ground maize were common ingredients in Blue Zones diets around the world. Wheat was not as important in ancient societies, and the grains they utilized contained less gluten than modern strains.
- Make vegetable soup with any leftover vegetables in your fridge by cutting them, frying them in olive oil and herbs, and then adding boiling water to cover. Simmer until the vegetables are tender, then season with salt & pepper to taste. Freeze what you don't eat right away in single or family-size containers, then reheat when you don't have time to prepare later in the week or month.

<u>**4. Sour on Bread**</u>

Sourdough or complete bread made with whole wheat should be used instead of regular bread.

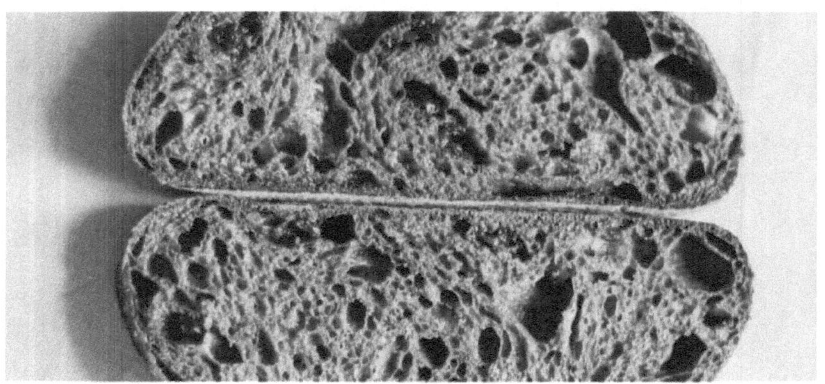

Bread has been consumed by humans for a minimum of 10,000 years. It is still a staple across three of the five blue zones. While it isn't frequently utilized for sandwiches, it does occur at most meals. However, what individuals in blue zones eat is not the same as the bread that the vast majority of North Americans consume. The majority of commercially available loaves begin with bleached white flour, which swiftly metabolizes into sugar. White bread provides few calories and raises insulin levels. White bread (together with glucose) actually represents the typical glycemic index value of 100, contrary to which all other foods are scored.

Ways you can accomplish it:

- If you're going to eat bread, make sure it's true sourdough bread from Ikaria. This slow-rising bread, also known as pain au levain, is baked with lactobacteria as a rising agent rather than commercial yeast.

- Try making sourdough bread from scratch using a genuine sourdough starter.
- Include sprouted grain bread in your Blue Zones diet. According to scientists, sprouting grains makes carbohydrates and proteins easier to digest. Sprouted breads also include more critical amino acids, minerals, and B vitamins than traditional whole-grain breads, as well as more useable iron. Sprouts are regarded to be part of the most nutritious foods, ounce for ounce.
- Full-grain rye or pumpernickel bread has a lower glycemic index than whole wheat bread. But have a look at the label. Avoid rye loaves using wheat flour as the first ingredient and instead, opt for rye bread with rye flour as the first ingredient. The majority of supermarket breads are not real rye breads.
- Select or create bread with seeds, nuts, dried fruits, and whole grains. Flaxseeds, as a whole food, add flavor, depth, texture, and health benefits.
- Look for coarse barley bread that has 75% to 80% whole barley kernels.
- In general, if you can roll a slice of bread into a ball, you should avoid it. Look for breads that are thick, dense, and made entirely of whole grains.

Consume up to three ounces of fish per day.

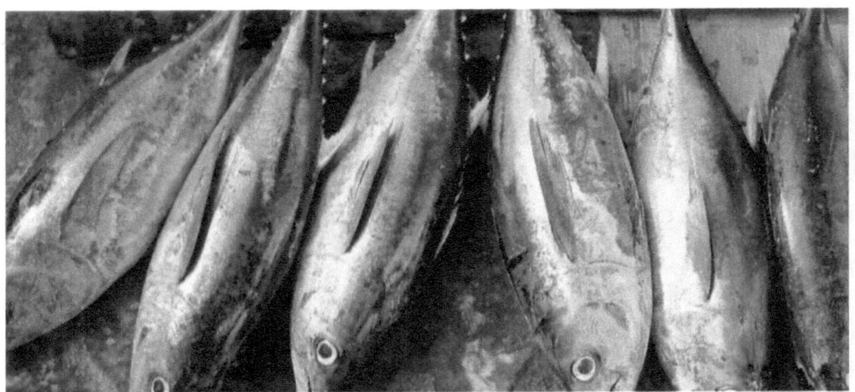

Consider three ounces to be the size of a deck of cards before cooking. Choose common and numerous fish that are not threatened by overfishing. The Adventist Health Study 2, which has followed 96,000 Americans since 2002, discovered that the persons who lived the longest did not eat meat or veganism. They were "pesco-vegetarians," or pescatarians, people who ate a plant-based diet with a modest amount of fish once or twice a week. Fish was a common part of everyday meals in other Blue Zones diets, eaten on average two to three times per week.

Ways you can accomplish it:

- Understand what three ounces of a larger fish, such as snapper or trout, or three ounces of a smaller fish, such as sardines or anchovies, looks like.

- Prefer mid-chain species such as trout, snapper, grouper, sardines, and anchovies. Avoid predator fish such as swordfish, sharks, and tuna if you want to imitate a Blue Zones diet. Avoid overfishing, such as Chilean sea bass.

- Avoid "farmed" fish because they are frequently raised in overcrowded quarters, necessitating the use of antibiotics, pesticides, and coloring.

6. Abstain from Meat

Limit your meat consumption to twice a week.

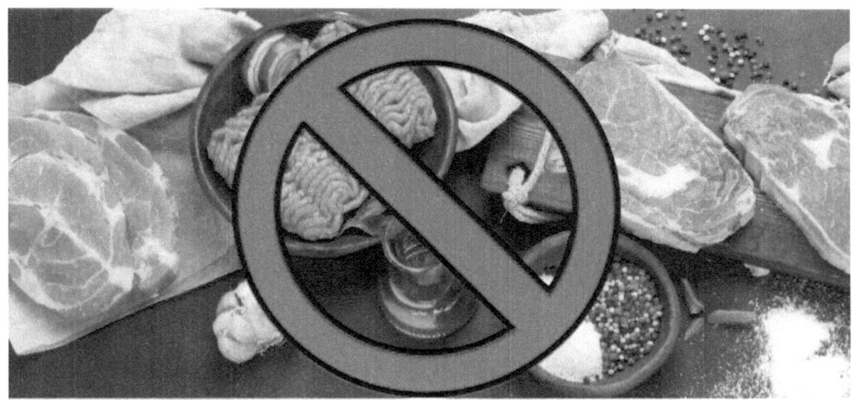

Consume meat twice a week or fewer, in quantities of no more than two ounces cooked. Choose free-range chicken and family-farmed hog or lamb over industrially reared meats. Hot dogs, luncheon meats, and sausages are examples of processed meats to avoid.

When meat intake was averaged throughout all blue zones, it was discovered that people ate small quantities of meat, roughly two ounces or less at a time, which was approximately five times per month. They splurged once a month, usually on grilled pig or goat. The usual Blue Zones diet does not include much meat or turkey.

The meat consumed in the blue zones is derived from free-roaming animals. These animals are not given hormones, pesticides, or antibiotics, and they are not subjected to the suffering of large feedlots.

Ways you can accomplish it:

- See what two ounces of cooked beef looks like: Half a chicken breast fillet or the flesh (without the skin) of a chicken leg before cooking, cut a pork or lamb chop or slice the size of a deck of cards.
- Avoid bringing in beef, hot dogs, luncheon meats, sausages, or other processed meats because they are not part of the Blue Zones diet.
- Look for plant-based alternatives to the meat that Americans are accustomed to having at the center of a meal. Try lightly sautéed tofu drizzled with olive oil, tempeh, or black bean or chickpea cakes.
- Set aside two days per week for meat or other animal-derived foods, and eat them solely on those days.
- Because restaurant meat portions are nearly four ounces or more, share meat entrées with another person or request a container ahead of time to carry half the meat amount home for later.

7. Eat Egg Occasionaly

Limit yourself to three eggs per week.

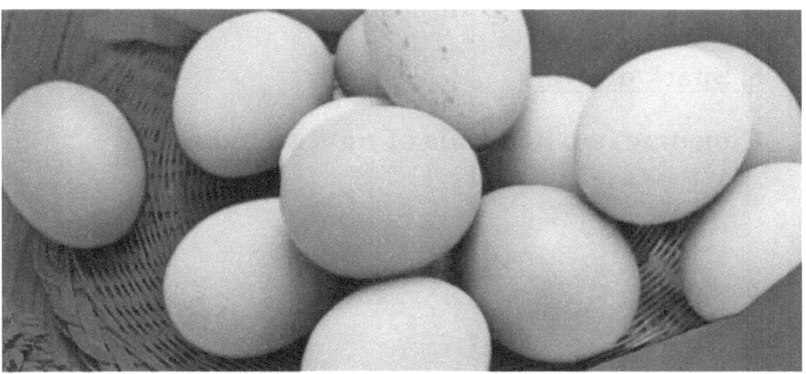

Eggs are part of the five Blue Zones eating habits, with people eating them two to four times per week on average. The egg, like meat protein, is a side dish that is eaten alongside a bigger piece of a whole-grain or other plant-based food component. Nicoyans fried an egg and served it with a corn tortilla and beans. In Okinawan soup, an egg is boiled. For breakfast, people in the Mediterranean Blue zones fried an egg with bread, nuts, and olives.

Eggs in the Blue Zones diet are produced by birds that are free to roam, consume a broad variety of natural foods, are not given hormones or antibiotics, and produce eggs that are naturally enriched in omega-3 fatty acids.

Ways you can accomplish it:

- Purchase only tiny eggs from pastured, cage-free birds.
- Add fruit or other plant-based items to a one-egg breakfast, such as whole-grain porridge or bread.

- As part of your Blue Zones diet, consider substituting scrambled tofu for eggs.

8. Snack on Nuts

Consume two handfuls of nuts each day.

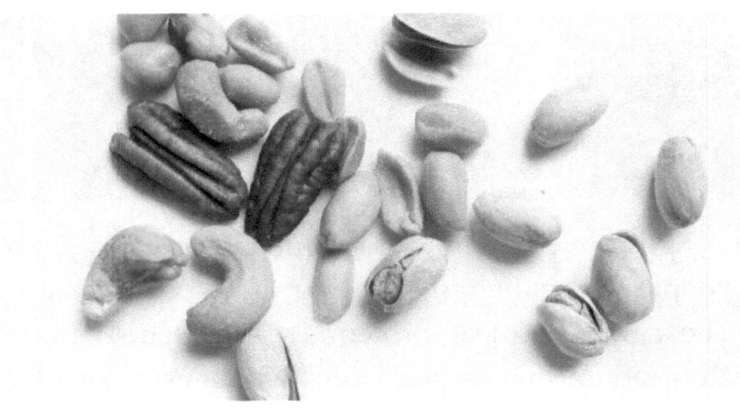

A handful of nuts equals around two ounces, which seems to be the typical amount of nuts consumed among blue zone centenarians. Here's how nuts are eaten in the different Blue Zones diets: Almonds are good in Ikaria and Sardinia, pistachios in Nicoya, and all nuts are well with Adventists. In accordance with the Adventist Health Study 2, nut eaters outlast non-nut eaters by two to three years on average.

Similarly, a recent Harvard study of 100,000 people tracked for 30 years discovered that nut eaters have a 20% lower mortality risk than non-nut eaters. Other studies demonstrate that eating nuts lowers the amount of "bad" LDL cholesterol from 9% to 20%, irrespective of the number of nuts eaten or the fat content. Copper, fiber, folate, vitamin E, and arginine, an amino acid, are all healthy elements in nuts.

Ways you can accomplish it:

- Keep nuts on hand for mid-morning or mid-afternoon snacks. Travel and vehicle journeys require modest packages.
- Incorporate nuts or other seeds into salads and soups.
- Keep a variety of nuts on hand to incorporate into your Blue Zones diet. Almonds (heavy in vitamin E and magnesium), peanuts (heavy in protein and folate, a B vitamin), Brazil nuts (heavy in selenium, a mineral thought to safeguard against cancers of the prostate), cashews (rich in magnesium), and walnuts (heavy in alpha-linoleic acid, the only omega-3 fat found in a plant-based food) are the best combination. All of these nuts will aid in cholesterol reduction.
- Include nuts as a protein source in your regular meals.
- Consume some nuts prior to a meal to lower your overall glycemic load.

<u>**9. Reduce Dairy**</u>

Reduce your intake of cow's milk and dairy products like cheese, cream, and butter.

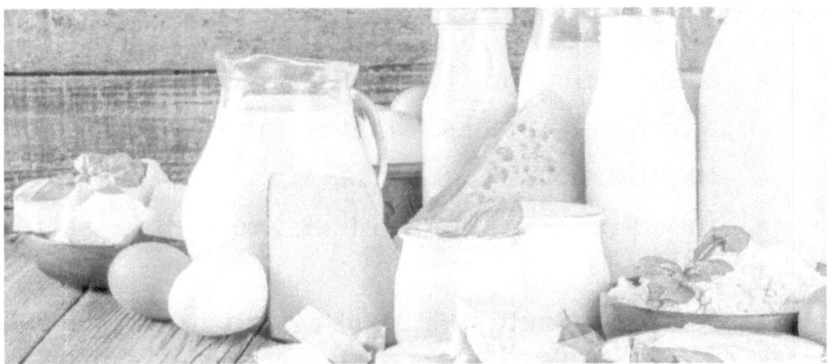

Except for Adventists, who consume eggs and dairy products, cow's milk plays no role in any Blue Zones diet. Dairy is a relative newcomer to the human diet, having been introduced between 8,000 and 10,000 years ago. Our digestive systems are not designed for anything made from milk (other than human milk), and we now know that up to 60% of people (sometimes inadvertently) have difficulties digesting lactose.

Ways you can accomplish it:

- As a dairy substitute, try unprocessed soy, coconut, or almond-based milk. Most have the same amount of protein as ordinary milk and typically taste just as nice or better.
- Cheese prepared from grass-fed goats or sheep will satisfy your periodic cheese cravings. Try pecorino sardo from Sardinia or Greek feta. Because they are

both rich, you only need a small amount to taste meals.

10. Be Completely Whole

Consume meals that are easily identified as such.

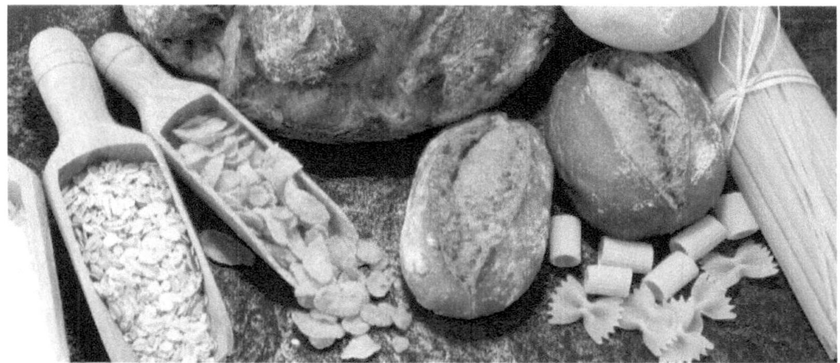

A "whole food" is also one that is prepared from a single ingredient, is uncooked, boiled, ground, or fermented, and is not excessively processed. (For example, tofu is little processed, whereas cheesy doodles and frozen sausage dogs are extensively processed.)

Humans traditionally eat the full meal in the world's blue zones and diets. They don't discard the yolk when making an egg-white omelet, nor do they strain the fat from their yogurt or juice the fiber-rich pulp from their fruits. They also do not enhance or add extra ingredients to their cuisine in order to affect the nutritional profile. They acquire what they need from nutrient-dense, fiber-rich whole foods rather than vitamins or other supplements. When they cook, they usually use a half dozen or so items that are simply combined together.

Ways you can accomplish it:

- Purchase items at market stalls for farmers or community-supported farms in your area.
- Avoid processed meals.
- Avoid eating foods that have been wrapped in plastic.
- Avoid foods that have more than five components.
- Stay away from ready-to-eat meals.
- Consume at least three Super Blue Foods per day (see list below). You don't have to eat a lot of these things. However, you will likely discover that these foods go a long way toward boosting your energy and sense of vitality, making you less tempted to go for the sugary, fatty, and processed foods that provide an instant (and brief) "fix."

The Blue Zones Beverage Guidelines

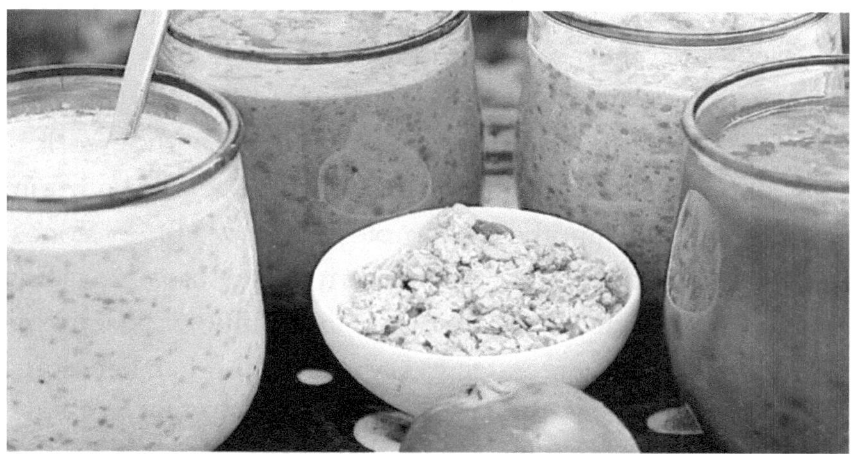

Drink coffee in the morning, tea in the afternoon, wine at 5 p.m., and water throughout the day. Never, ever consume soda pop, even diet soda.

People in blue zones drank water, coffee, tea, and wine with few exceptions. Period. (Most blue zone centenarians had never heard of soda pop, which accounts for roughly half of America's sugar intake.) Each has a compelling argument.

- **Water:** Seven glasses of water every day is officially recommended by Adventists. They cite research that suggests that staying hydrated improves blood flow and reduces the risk of a blood clot. There is an additional benefit, in my opinion: when people drink water, they are not consuming a sugar-laden drink (soda, Energizers, and fruit juices) or an unnaturally sweetened drink, a lot of which are potentially harmful.

- **Coffee:** Sardinians, Ikarians, and Nicoyans all consume a lot of coffee. According to research, coffee consumption is associated with a lower risk of dementia and Parkinson's disease. Furthermore, coffee is often shade grown in the world's blue zones, which benefits birds and the environment — yet another example of how Blue Zones' diet patterns reflect a concern for the broader picture.
- **Tea:** Tea is consumed in all blue zones. Okinawans drink green tea every day, and it has been proven to reduce the risk of cardiovascular disease and various malignancies. Ikarians consume drinks made from rosemary, wild sage, and dandelion, all of which have anti-inflammatory qualities.
- **Red Wine:** Those who drink in moderation survive those who do not. (This is not to say you ought to begin to drink if you don't already.) Most blue zones consume between one and three cups of red wine every day, usually with food and with company. Wine has been shown to aid the body's absorption of plant-based antioxidants, making it an excellent addition to a Blue Zones diet. These advantages could be attributed to resveratrol, a red wine-specific antioxidant. However, it is possible that a small amount of alcohol at the final hour of the day relieves stress, which is beneficial to general health. In any event, consuming more than two to three glasses per day for women and men, respectively, is harmful to their health. Having more than one drink

each day increases the risk of developing breast cancer in women.

Ways you can accomplish it:

- Preserve a full water bottle by your bed and at your desk or workplace.
- You are welcome to begin the day with a cup of coffee. Coffee is gently sweetened and consumed black, without cream, in the Blue Zones diets.
- Avoid coffee after mid-afternoon because caffeine might interfere with sleep (centenarians, by the way, sleep an average of eight hours every night).
- Drink green tea all day; it contains roughly 25% as much caffeine as coffee and delivers a continual stream of antioxidants.
- Experiment with herbal teas like rosemary, oregano, or sage.
- Lightly sweeten drinks with honey and store in a pitcher in the fridge for quick access in hot weather.
- Never bring soft drinks into your home.

Research has validated several fundamental principles of the Blues Zones diet. These include:

- A diet higher in plant-based foods was linked to a lower risk of heart disease death overall, as per a study published in the August 2019 issue of the Journal of the American Heart Association.
- A March 2021 study published in The Journal of Nutrition suggests that eating more whole grains may reduce your risk of pancreatic cancer.

The U.S. dietary guidelines for whole grains, which include consuming at least three servings a day, are cited by the Blue Zones diet. Additionally, eating a lot of beans may lower your chance of developing several cancers.

- Eating a Mediterranean-style diet, such as the Blue Zones diet, may also change your microbiome in a way that will help you age more cognitively and less fragile.
- Studies suggest that increasing your intake of nuts, as advised by the Blue Zones diet, may lower your risk of cardiovascular disease.
- An all-encompassing review that was published in the journal Nutrients in July 2020 suggested that eating a diet high in plants and whole foods could considerably lower your risk of type 2 diabetes. Conversely, diets heavy in processed meat and sugar, or in beverages sweetened with artificial sugar, markedly raised the risk of metabolic illness.

- Consuming fruits, vegetables, whole grains, and fiber may promote deeper, more restful sleep and reduce the symptoms of insomnia.
- According to a March 2021 study published in Antioxidants, polyphenols—healthy substances present in plant-based foods—may contribute to a longer life by delaying the onset of age-related disorders including diabetes and cardiovascular disease.
- The Blue Zones diet aims to improve your quality of life rather than aid in weight loss. However, this healthy eating approach may result in weight loss as a side effect. Whole foods, according to Dr. Rajagopal, "tend to have fewer calories than processed forms of carbohydrates, protein, or fats," and are the cornerstone of the diet. As a result, "people who follow this diet tend to maintain a healthier weight because they consume fewer calories overall."

PROS AND CONS OF BLUE ZONES DIET

The Blue Zones diet is a component of a larger way of living that includes emphasizes stress reduction, natural movement, purposeful living, and fostering relationships with loved ones and the community. All of the heart-healthy, cancer-fighting, and other health benefits mentioned above are provided by the Blue Zones diet. Additionally, we have noted that:

- The Blue Zones diet doesn't need you to purchase any unique goods or services; you can come across these foods at farmers' markets and supermarkets.
- No tedious counting or measuring is required. You eat in accordance with your level of hunger and quit when you're eighty percent full. Calorie and macro tracking is not required.

Does the Blue Zones diet have any drawbacks, then? We looked into the nutrition and found nothing wrong, but switching from what you are eating now can take some time and work, particularly if you are a quick eater. It's possible that cooking will be more difficult than it is now.

"There may be a significant shift from your typical eating habits, which requires adaptation," advises Cassetty. You have to allow yourself time to experiment with different cuisines and cooking techniques.

According to Rajagopal, "learning about the various components and how to incorporate them into your lifestyle takes time." Rather than completely changing your diet at once, she suggests expanding on the foods that are currently a part of the Blue Zones diet and making one or two more changes at a time.

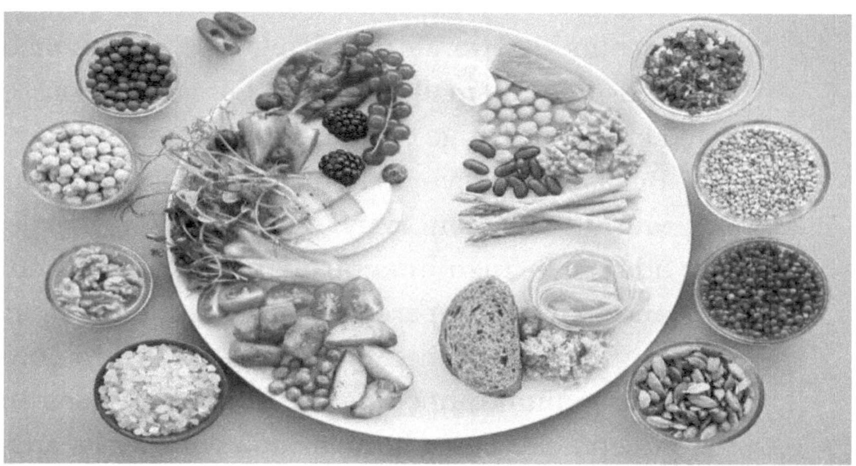

4 to Always Eat

Remembering four food types may be an easier point of entry than remembering all of the Blue Zones diet foods. This is our list.

1. **100% Whole Wheat Bread:** We reasoned that it could be toasted in the morning and then used to make a nutritious sandwich for lunch. While it may not be the ideal longevity meal, it may assist in eliminating white bread from the diet and be an important step toward a healthier Blue Zones diet for most Americans.

2. **Nuts:** We know that nut eaters outlive non-nut eaters. Nuts come in a variety of flavors and are high in nutrients and healthy fats that satisfy your hunger. A two-ounce mix of nuts (roughly a

handful) is the ideal snack. You should ideally keep tiny two-ounce containers on hand. Because the oils in nuts deteriorate (oxidize), it is recommended to consume in small amounts. Larger portions can be kept in the fridge or freezer for a few months.

3. **Beans:** I believe that all types of beans are the world's best longevity foods. They're inexpensive, adaptable, high in antioxidants, vitamins, and fiber, and may be prepared to taste excellent. It's ideal to buy dry beans because they're easier to cook, but low-sodium canned beans in non-BPA cans are also acceptable. Learn how to cook with beans and stock up on them, and you'll be well on your way to living further with a Blue Zones diet.

4. **Your Favorite Fruit:** Purchase a lovely fruit dish, set it in the center of your kitchen area (either the work surface, center location, or table — wherever there is the most activity), and illuminate it. According to research, we eat what we see, so if chips remain in easy access, we'll consume them. However, if you enjoy a certain fruit and keep it in plain sight at all times, you will eat much more of it and be healthier as a result. Avoid the expense of buying a fruit that you believe you should eat but actually dislike.

4 to Always Avoid

1. **Sugar-Sweetened Beverages:** Harvard's Willett estimates that empty calories and liquid sugar in sodas and packaged juices account for 50% of America's caloric gain. Would you eat your cereal

with ten tablespoons of sugar? Most likely not. But that's how much sugar you get from a 12-ounce can of soda pop on average.

2. **Salty Snacks:** We spend roughly $6 billion each year on potato chips, the food most strongly associated with obesity (but fried pig rinds are closing in fast). Almost all chips and crackers contain a lot of salt, preservatives, and highly processed carbohydrates that quickly turn into sugar. They've also been meticulously crafted to be maximally crispy and flavorful, with a seductive tongue feel. In other words, they're designed to be unstoppable. So, how do you deal with them? You should not have them inside your home!

3. **Processed Meats:** A current gold-standard epidemiology study monitored more than 500,000 people for decades and discovered that those who ate the most sausages, salami, bacon, lunch meats, and other extremely processed meats had the highest incidences of cancer and heart disease. Once again, the threat is dual. These meat products include carcinogenic nitrates and other preservatives. They perform the job, however, and the products are well preserved, which means that meat that has been processed is readily available on the shelf at home or in the supermarket, right there for munching or a quick meal—something that Blue Zones households and diets do not have.

4. **Packaged Sweets:** Cookies, candy bars, muffins, granola bars, and even energy bars, like salty snacks,

pack a punch of insulin-spiking sweets. We're all genetically predisposed to seek sweets, so we immediately want to satisfy our hunger by tearing open a package of cookies and eating in. Lessons from the Blue Zones diet would suggest that if you intend to bake some cookies or a cake and keep them around, that's fine. If you want to treat yourself to a baked good from your local bakery, that's acceptable. But don't keep any sugary food in your pantry.

List of foods

Vegetables

- Fennel
- Potatoes
- Shiitake mushrooms
- Squash
- Sweet potatoes
- Kombu (seaweed)
- Wild greens
- Wakame (seaweed)
- Tomatoes
- Yams Zucchini
- Cucumbers
- Eggplant
- Onions
- Garlic

Fruits

- Lemons
- Papayas
- Avocados
- Pejivalles (peach palms)
- Plantains
- Bananas
- Bitter melons

Beans (Legumes)

- Chickpeas
- Black beans
- Fava beans
- Black-eyed peas
- Kidney beans
- Cannellini beans
- Pinto beans
- Edamame

Grains

- Brown rice
- Farro
- Barley
- Quinoa
- Oats
- Whole wheat pasta
- Bulgur
- Millet

Nuts and Seeds

- Almonds
- Walnuts
- Chia seeds
- Flaxseeds
- Sunflower seeds
- Pumpkin see

Lean Protein

- Tofu
- Tempeh
- Lean poultry (chicken, turkey)
- Fish (salmon, trout, sardines)
- Beans and legumes (as mentioned above)
- Eggs

Dairy

- Feta cheese
- Pecorino cheese

Added Oils

- Olive oil

Beverages

- Coffee
- Green tea
- Red wine
- Water

Sweeteners and Seasonings

- Garlic
- Honey
- Mediterranean herbs
- Milk thistle
- Turmeric

28-DAY MEAL PLAN

Day 1:

- **Breakfast:** Blue Zones Cornmeal Waffles
- **Lunch:** Sardinian Herbed Lentil Minestrone
- **Dinner:** Southwestern Quinoa Burgers

Day 2:

- **Breakfast:** Acai Bowl with Blueberries, Granola, and Coconut
- **Lunch:** Greek Salad with Feta Cheese and Olives
- **Dinner:** Vegetarian Spaghetti Bolognese

Day 3:

- **Breakfast:** Quinoa and Black Bean Breakfast Burrito
- **Lunch:** Mexican Pozole Verde
- **Dinner:** Gullah Shrimp and Grits

Day 4:

- **Breakfast:** Chia Seed Pudding combined with Nuts and Berries
- **Lunch:** Roasted Broccoli with Lemon and Parmesan Cheese
- **Dinner:** Cajun Blackened Salmon

Day 5:

- **Breakfast:** Tofu Scramble with Mushrooms and Spinach
- **Lunch:** Tuscan Kale Salad with White Beans and Lemon Vinaigrette
- **Dinner:** Key Lime Pie

Day 6:

- **Breakfast:** Boiled Eggs (boiled) combined with Everything but the Bagel Seasoning
- **Lunch:** Southern Coleslaw
- **Dinner:** Lemon Bars

Day 7:

- **Breakfast:** Smoothie with Spinach, Banana, and Berries
- **Lunch:** Gullah Gumbo
- **Dinner:** Chocolate Chip Cookies

Day 8:

- **Breakfast:** Acai Bowl with Blueberries, Granola, and Coconut

- **Lunch:** Southwestern Black Bean Salad
- **Dinner:** Northwest Salmon Chowder

Day 9:

- **Breakfast:** Chia Seed Pudding combined with Nuts and Berries
- **Lunch:** Roasted Brussels Sprouts with Bacon and Balsamic Vinegar
- **Dinner:** Peanut Butter Cookies

Day 10:

- **Breakfast:** Blue Zones Cornmeal Waffles
- **Lunch:** Greek Salad combined with Olives and Feta Cheese
- **Dinner:** Sardinian Herbed Lentil Minestrone

Day 11:

- **Breakfast:** Tofu Scramble with Mushrooms and Spinach
- **Lunch:** Louisiana Gumbo
- **Dinner:** Fresh Fruit Salad with Coconut Yogurt and Honey

Day 12:

- **Breakfast:** Quinoa and Black Bean Breakfast Burrito
- **Lunch:** Tuscan Kale Salad with White Beans and Lemon Vinaigrette
- **Dinner:** Dark Chocolate Avocado Mousse

Day 13:

- **Breakfast:** Boiled Eggs (boiled) combined with Everything but the Bagel Seasoning
- **Lunch:** Mediterranean Lentil Soup
- **Dinner:** Apple Crisp

Day 14:

- **Breakfast:** Acai Bowl with Blueberries, Granola, and Coconut
- **Lunch:** Greek Salad combined with Olives and Feta Cheese
- **Dinner:** Lentil Burgers on Whole-Wheat Buns with Sweet Potato Fries

Day 15:

- **Breakfast:** Smoothie with Spinach, Banana, and Berries
- **Lunch:** Mexican Pozole Verde
- **Dinner:** Baked Apples with Cinnamon and Sugar

Day 16:

- **Breakfast:** Tofu Scramble with Mushrooms and Spinach
- **Lunch:** Sardinian Herbed Lentil Minestrone
- **Dinner:** Southwest Quinoa Burgers

Day 17:

- **Breakfast:** Lemon Bars
- **Lunch:** Roasted Broccoli with Lemon and Parmesan Cheese
- **Dinner:** Key Lime Pie

Day 18:

- **Breakfast:** Boiled Eggs (boiled) combined with Everything but the Bagel Seasoning
- **Lunch:** Southwestern Black Bean Salad
- **Dinner:** Clam Chowder with Milk, Potatoes, and Clams

Day 19:

- **Breakfast:** Dark Chocolate Avocado Mousse
- **Lunch:** Roasted Brussels Sprouts with Bacon and Balsamic Vinegar
- **Dinner:** Peanut Butter Cookies

Day 20:

- **Breakfast:** Acai Bowl with Blueberries, Granola, and Coconut
- **Lunch:** Gullah Gumbo
- **Dinner:** Swedish Meatballs

Day 21:

- **Breakfast:** Smoothie with Spinach, Banana, and Berries
- **Lunch:** Mediterranean Lentil Soup
- **Dinner:** Fruit Sorbet with Mint and Lime

Day 22:

- **Breakfast:** Key Lime Pie
- **Lunch:** Greek Salad combined with Olives and Feta Cheese

- **Dinner:** Pueblo Green Chile Stew

Day 23:

- **Breakfast:** Quinoa and Black Bean Breakfast Burrito
- **Lunch:** Dark Chocolate Avocado Mousse
- **Dinner:** Hmong Spring Rolls

Day 24:

- **Breakfast:** Tofu Scramble with Mushrooms and Spinach
- **Lunch:** Roasted Cauliflower with Parmesan Cheese
- **Dinner:** Salmon with Roasted Vegetables and Lemon Aioli

Day 25:

- **Breakfast:** Acai Bowl with Blueberries, Granola, and Coconut
- **Lunch:** Mexican Pozole Verde
- **Dinner:** Oatmeal Cookies with Raisins and Nuts

Day 26:

- **Breakfast:** Boiled Eggs (boiled) combined with Everything but the Bagel Seasoning
- **Lunch:** Southern Coleslaw
- **Dinner:** Baked Apples with Cinnamon and Sugar

Day 27:

- **Breakfast:** Smoothie with Spinach, Banana, and Berries
- **Lunch:** Northwest Salmon Chowder

- **Dinner:** Peanut Butter Cookies

Day 28:

- **Breakfast:** Blue Zones Cornmeal Waffles
- **Lunch:** Gullah Shrimp and Grits
- **Dinner:** Fresh Fruit Salad with Coconut Yogurt and Honey

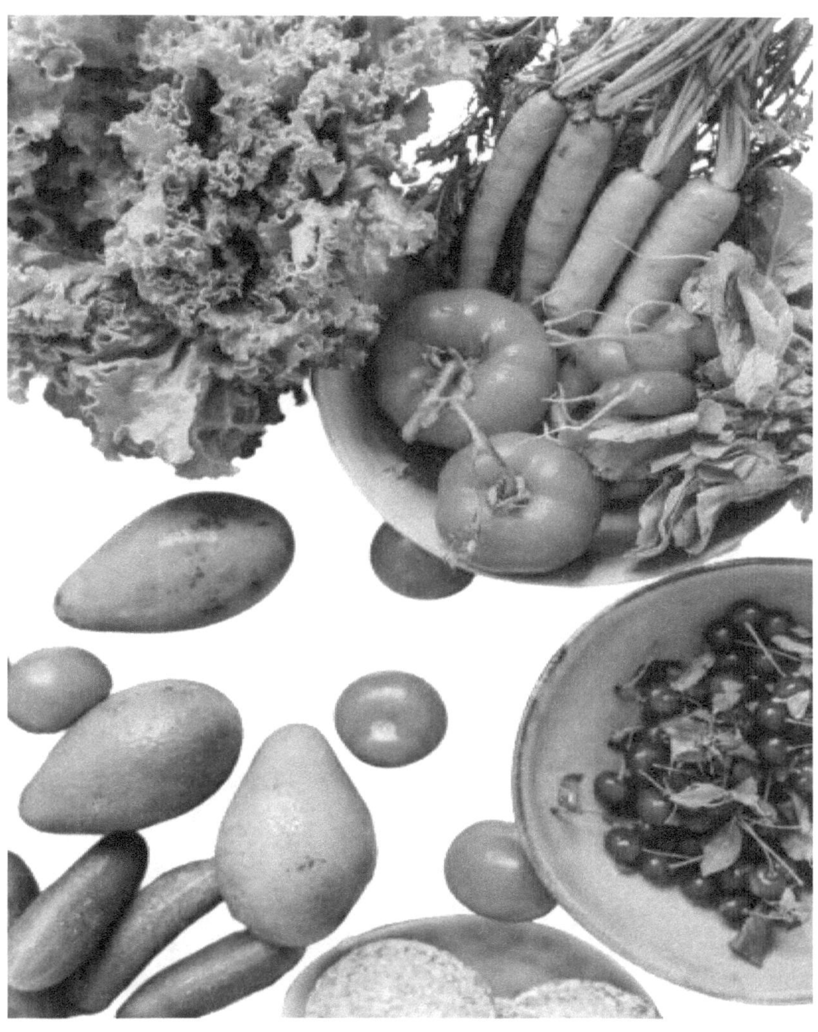

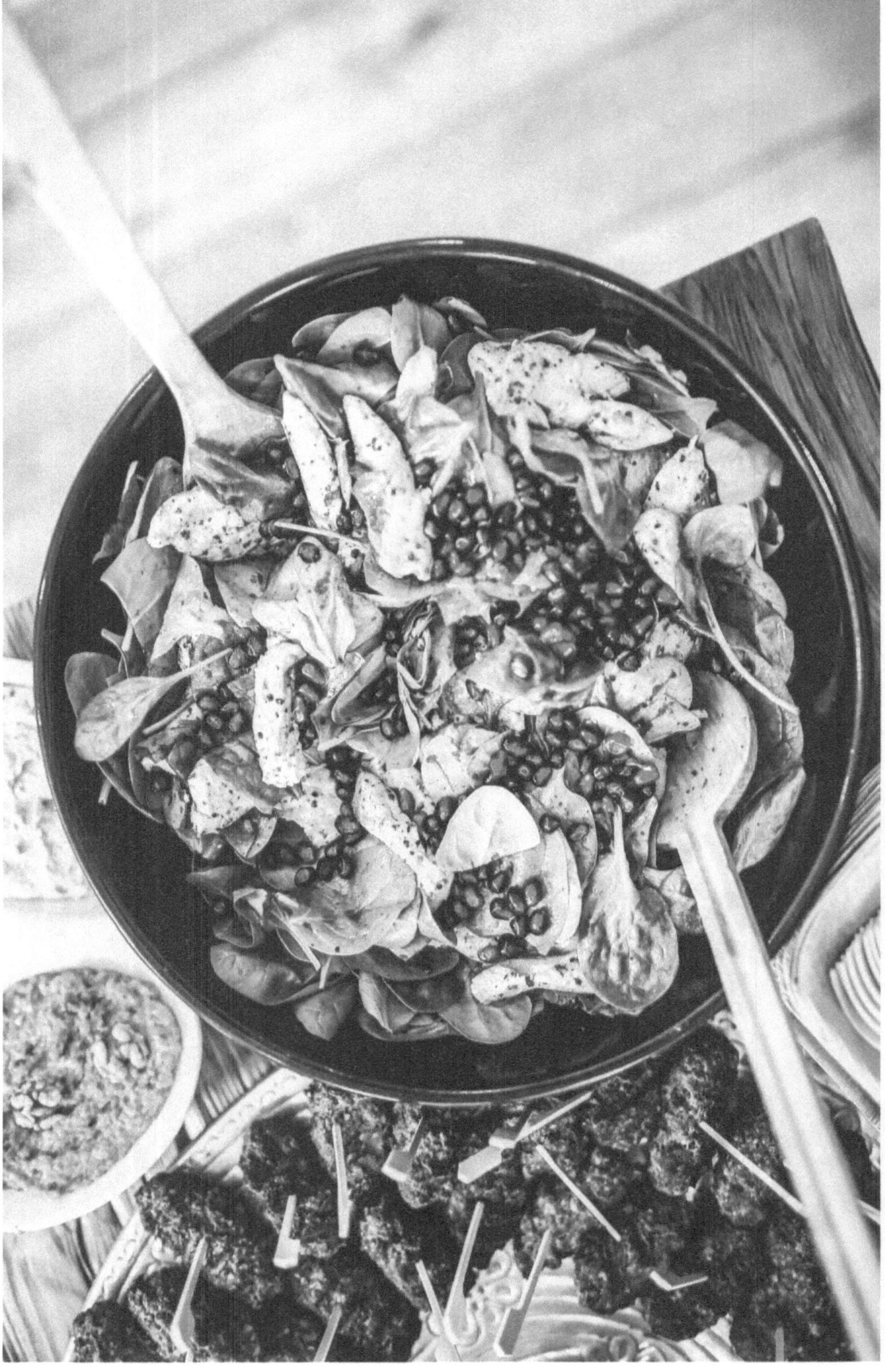

CHAPTER 2: HEALTHY DELICIOUS RECIPES

BREAKFAST RECIPES

Blue Zones Cornmeal Waffles

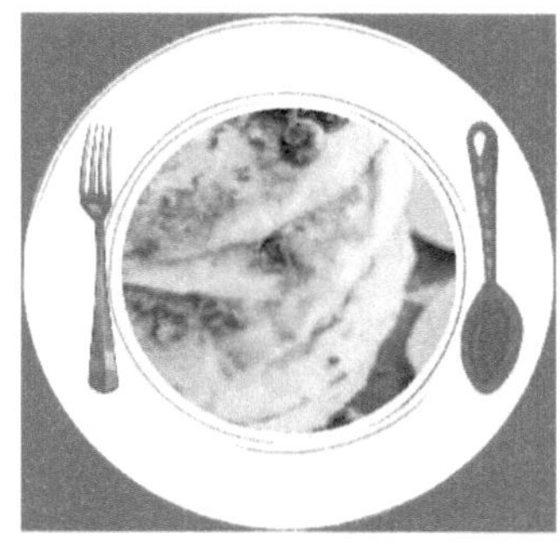

- **Serving Size:** 2 waffles

- **Prep Time:** 15 minutes

Ingredients:

- 1 cup cornmeal
- 1 cup whole wheat flour
- 2 tsp baking powder
- 1/2 tsp salt
- 2 tbsp honey or maple syrup
- 2 cups plant-based milk (e.g., almond, soy)
- 2 tbsp of melted coconut oil or canola oil

Instructions:

1. In a mixing bowl, combine the cornmeal, whole wheat flour, baking powder, and salt.
2. In a separate bowl, whisk together the honey or maple syrup, plant-based milk, and oil.
3. Add the dry ingredients to the wet ingredients and stir until it is evenly combined.
4. Waffle irons should be preheated and lightly oiled.
5. Pour the waffle batter into the iron and cook according to the manufacturer's instructions until golden brown.
6. Serve the waffles with your choice of fresh berries or a drizzle of honey or maple syrup.

Nutrient Information (per serving, without toppings):

- Calories: Approximately 320-350
- Protein: 7-9 grams
- Fat: 7-9 grams
- Carbohydrates: 60-70 grams
- Fiber: 6-8 grams

Acai Bowl with Blueberries, Granola, and Coconut

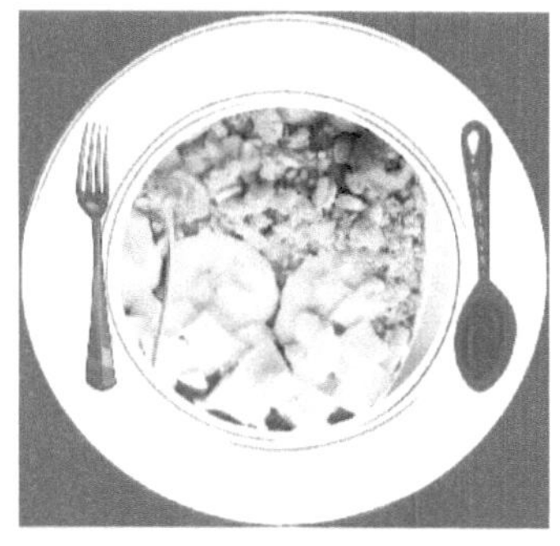

- **Serving Size:** 1 bowl
- **Prep Time:** 10 minutes

Ingredients:

- 1 packet frozen acai puree
- 1/2 cup frozen blueberries
- 1/2 banana
- 1/2 cup plant-based milk
- Toppings: Granola, shredded coconut, fresh blueberries, sliced banana, and a drizzle of honey (optional)

Instructions:

1. In a blender, combine the acai puree, frozen blueberries, banana, and plant-based milk.
2. Blend until smooth and creamy.
3. Gently pour the acai mixture into a basin.
4. Top with granola, shredded coconut, fresh blueberries, sliced banana, and a drizzle of honey if desired.

Nutrient Information (per serving, without optional honey):

- Calories: Approximately 350-400
- Protein: 4-6 grams
- Fat: 15-20 grams
- Carbohydrates: 50-60 grams
- Fiber: 10-12 grams

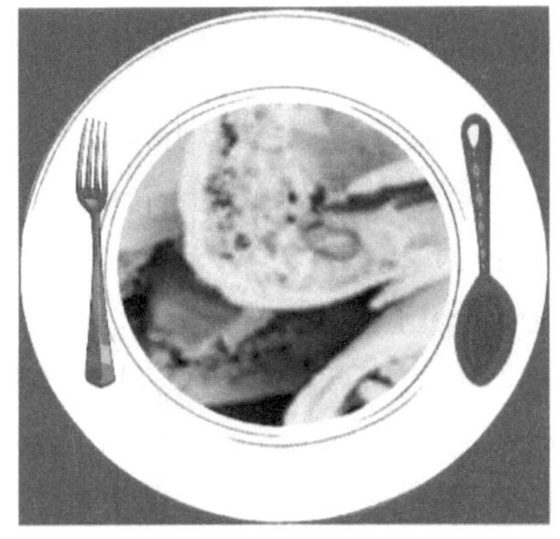

Quinoa and Black Bean Breakfast Burrito

- **Serving Size:** 1 burrito
- **Prep Time:** 20 minutes

Ingredients:

- 1/2 cup cooked quinoa
- 1/2 cup of black beans (canned), washed and drained
- 1/4 cup diced tomatoes
- 1/4 cup diced bell peppers
- 2 big-sized eggs (or tofu for vegan)

- 1/4 tsp cumin
- Salt and pepper to taste
- Whole-grain tortilla

Instructions:

1. In a skillet, sauté the diced tomatoes and bell peppers until tender.
2. Add the cooked quinoa and black beans to the skillet and heat through.
3. In a separate pan, scramble the eggs (or tofu) with cumin, salt, and pepper.
4. Assemble the burrito by placing the quinoa and black bean mixture, followed by the scrambled eggs (or tofu) onto a whole-grain tortilla.
5. Roll the tortilla into a burrito, folding in the sides.

Nutrient Information (per serving):

- Calories: Approximately 350-400
- Protein: 15-20 grams
- Fat: 8-10 grams
- Carbohydrates: 50-60 grams
- Fiber: 10-12 grams

Chia Seed Pudding combined with Nuts and Berries

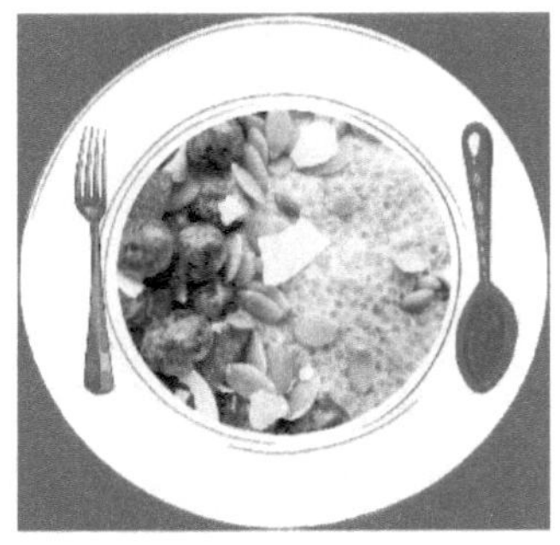

- **Serving Size:** 1 bowl
- **Prep Time:** 5 minutes (plus the time for chilling)

Ingredients:

- 2 tbsp chia seeds
- 1/2 cup plant-based milk
- 1/2 tsp honey or maple syrup
- Fresh berries (e.g., strawberries, blueberries)
- Chopped nuts (e.g., almonds, walnuts)

Instructions:

1. In an average-sized bowl, combine together the chia seeds, plant-based milk, and honey or maple syrup.
2. Stir thoroughly to make sure the chia seeds are dispersed equally.
3. Refrigerate the mixture for at least 2 hours or overnight, allowing it to thicken.
4. Top with fresh berries and chopped nuts before serving.

Nutrient Information (per serving, without toppings):

- Calories: Approximately 180-220
- Protein: 4-6 grams
- Fat: 8-10 grams
- Carbohydrates: 15-20 grams
- Fiber: 6-8 grams

Tofu Scramble with Mushrooms and Spinach

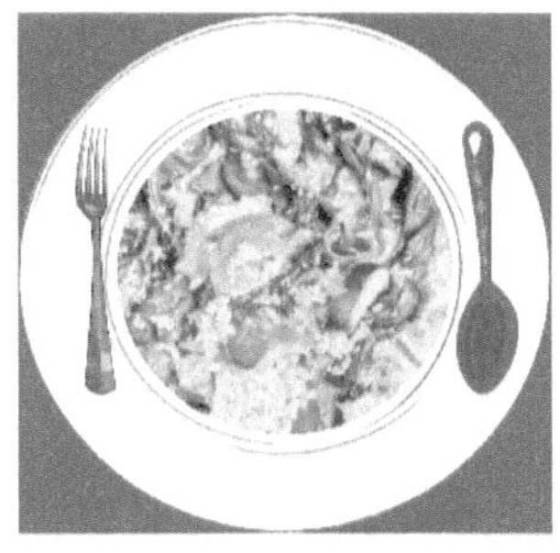

- **Serving Size:** 1 serving
- **Prep Time:** 15 minutes

Ingredients:

- 1/2 cup firm tofu, crumbled
- 1/2 cup sliced mushrooms
- 1 cup fresh spinach
- 1/4 cup diced onions
- 1/4 tsp turmeric (for color)
- Salt and pepper to taste

Instructions:

1. In a skillet, sauté the diced onions until they become translucent.
2. Put the sliced mushrooms and cook well until they start to release their moisture and become soft.
3. Stir in the crumbled tofu and turmeric, and cook for a few minutes, mimicking scrambled eggs.
4. Include fresh spinach to the pan and cook until shriveled.
5. Add pepper and salt as seasoning to your preferred taste.

Nutrient Information (per serving):

- Calories: Approximately 200-250
- Protein: 12-15 grams
- Fat: 10-12 grams
- Carbohydrates: 10-12 grams
- Fiber: 4-6 grams

Hmong Spring Rolls

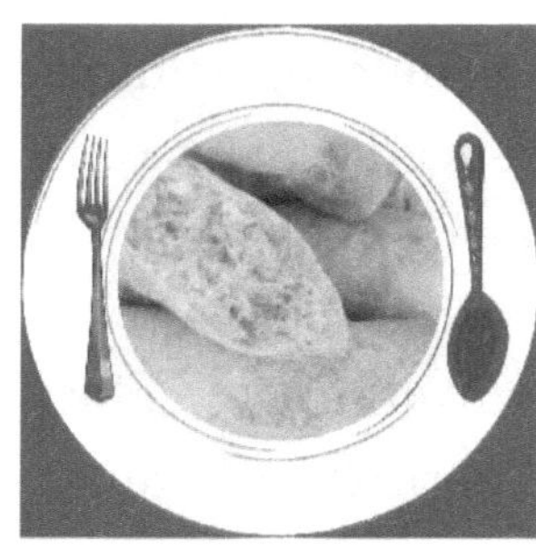

- **Serving Size:** 2 spring rolls
- **Prep Time:** 30 minutes

Ingredients:

- 4 rice paper wrappers
- 1 cup cooked vermicelli noodles
- 1 cup cooked shrimp, sliced in half lengthwise
- 1 cup fresh herbs (e.g., cilantro, mint, basil)
- 1 cup lettuce leaves
- 1/2 cup bean sprouts
- For dipping, use peanut sauce and hoisin sauce

Instructions:

1. Prepare a shallow dish of warm water.
2. Dip a rice paper wrapper into the warm water to soften it. Place it on a clean surface.
3. Layer vermicelli noodles, shrimp, fresh herbs, lettuce leaves, and bean sprouts in the center of the wrapper.
4. Fold in the sides of the wrapper, then roll it up tightly, similar to a burrito.
5. Repeat the process by using the remaining ingredients and wrappers.
6. Gently serve the spring rolls alongside with hoisin sauce and peanut sauce for dipping.

Nutrient Information (per 2 spring rolls, without dipping sauce):

- Calories: Approximately 150-200
- Protein: 10-12 grams
- Fat: 1-2 grams
- Carbohydrates: 30-35 grams
- Fiber: 2-3 grams

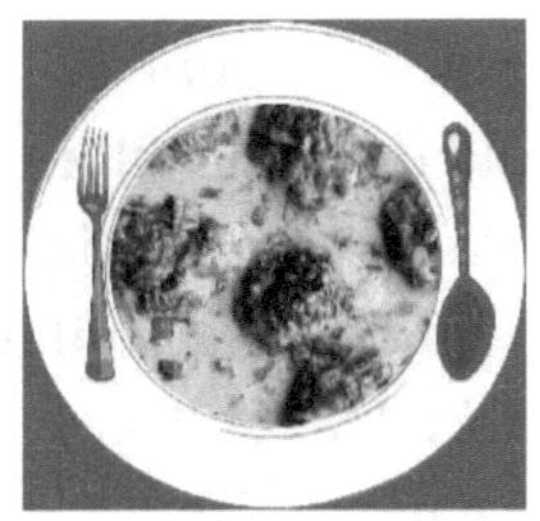

- **Serving Size:** 4-5 meatballs
- **Prep Time:** 25 minutes + 20 minutes cooking time

Ingredients:

For the meatballs:

- 1/2 lb ground beef
- 1/2 lb ground lamb
- 1/2 cup breadcrumbs
- 1/4 cup milk
- 1 small onion, finely chopped
- 1/2 tsp allspice
- 1/2 tsp salt
- 1/4 tsp black pepper

For the gravy:

- 1 cup beef broth
- 1/2 cup heavy cream
- 2 tbsp butter
- 2 tbsp all-purpose flour

Lingonberry sauce for serving (optional)

Instructions:

1. In an average-sized bowl, combine togetherground beef, ground lamb, breadcrumbs, milk, finely chopped onion, allspice, salt, and black pepper.
2. Form the mixture into small meatballs.
3. Heat up the pan over moderate-high flame and cook the meatballs until they are browned and cooked through.
4. In the same pan, melt butter and stir in all-purpose flour to create a roux.
5. Pour in beef broth and heavy cream, stirring until the gravy thickens.
6. Serve the meatballs with the gravy and lingonberry sauce, if desired.

Nutrient Information (per 4-5 meatballs, without lingonberry sauce):

- Calories: Approximately 250-300
- Protein: 15-20 grams
- Fat: 15-20 grams
- Carbohydrates: 10-15 grams
- Fiber: 1-2 grams

- Serving Size: 2 hard-boiled eggs
- Prep Time: 12-15 minutes

Ingredients:

- 2 big-sized eggs
- Homemade or store-bought Everything But the Bagel Seasoning

Instructions:

1. Put the eggs in a saucepan and pour water to cover them.
2. Bring the water to a boil, then reduce the heat and simmer for 9-12 minutes.
3. Drain the hot water and transfer the eggs to a bowl of ice water to cool.
4. Remove the shell of the eggs after they've cooled.
5. Sprinkle the hard-boiled eggs with Everything But the Bagel Seasoning.

Nutrient Information (per serving):

- Calories: Approximately 140-160
- Protein: 12-14 grams
- Fat: 10-12 grams
- Carbohydrates: 1-2 grams
- Fiber: Less than 1 gram

Chia Pudding with Coconut Milk and Mango

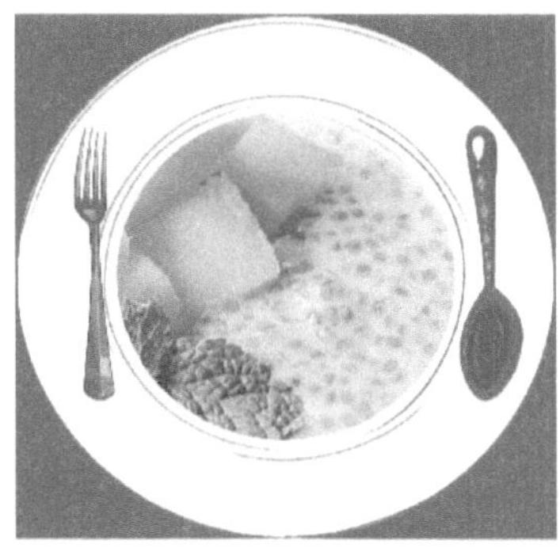

- **Serving Size:** 1 serving
- **Prep Time:** 5 minutes (plus time of chilling)

Ingredients:

- 2 tablespoons chia seeds
- 1/2 cup coconut milk
- 1/2 cup diced mango
- 1 tablespoon of maple syrup or honey (if desired)
- Fresh mint leaves for garnish

Instructions:

1. In a moderate-sized bowl, combine chia seeds and coconut milk.
2. Sweeten with honey or maple syrup if desired.
3. Chill the mixture in the refrigerator for a few hours or overnight until it thickens.
4. Top with diced mango and garnish with fresh mint leaves.

Nutrient Information (per serving, without sweetener):

- Calories: Approximately 250-300

- Protein: 5-7 grams
- Fat: 15-20 grams
- Carbohydrates: 25-30 grams
- Fiber: 10-12 grams

Smoothie with Spinach, Banana, and Berries

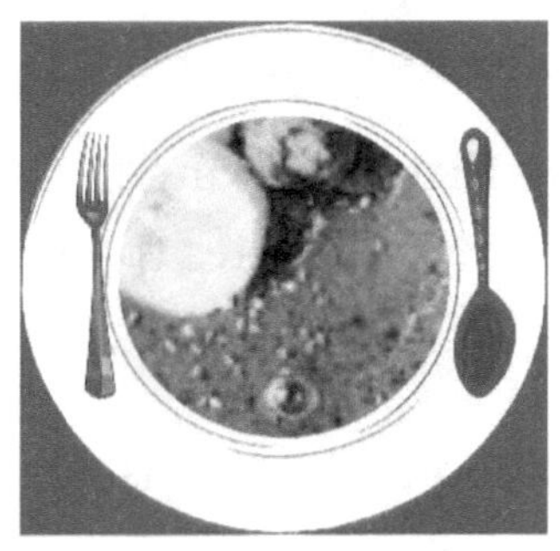

- **Serving Size:** 1 smoothie
- **Prep Time:** 5 minutes

Ingredients:

- 1 cup fresh spinach leaves
- 1 ripe banana
- 1/2 a cup of mixed berries, such as strawberries and blueberries
- 1/2 cup Greek yogurt
- 1/2 cup water or coconut water
- 1 tablespoon honey (optional)

Instructions:

1. Place spinach, banana, mixed berries, Greek yogurt, and water in a blender.

2. Add honey for sweetness if desired.
3. Blend until smooth.

Nutrient Information (per serving, without honey):

- Calories: Approximately 200-250
- Protein: 10-12 grams
- Fat: 2-3 grams
- Carbohydrates: 40-45 grams
- Fiber: 7-9 grams

Sardinian Herbed Lentil Minestrone

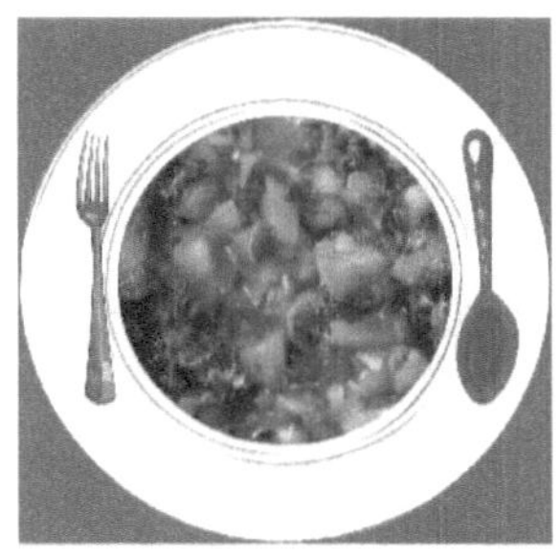

- **Serving Size:** 1 bowl
- **Prep Time:** 30 minutes

Ingredients:

- 1/2 cup of readily dried lentils (brown/green)
- 4 cups vegetable broth
- 1 cup diced tomatoes
- 1/2 cup diced zucchini

- 1/2 cup diced carrots
- 1/2 cup diced celery
- 1/2 cup diced onions
- 2 cloves garlic, minced
- 1 tsp dried Italian herbs (e.g., oregano, basil, thyme)
- Salt and pepper to taste

Instructions:

1. In a big-sized pot, sauté the diced onions and garlic until fragrant and translucent.
2. Add lentils, vegetable broth, diced tomatoes, zucchini, carrots, celery, and dried Italian herbs to the pot.
3. Bring the mixture to a boil, then reduce heat and simmer for about 20-25 minutes until the lentils and vegetables are tender.
4. Add pepper and salt as seasoning to your preferred taste.

Nutrient Information (per serving):

- Calories: Approximately 200-250
- Protein: 10-12 grams
- Fat: 1-2 grams
- Carbohydrates: 40-45 grams
- Fiber: 10-12 grams

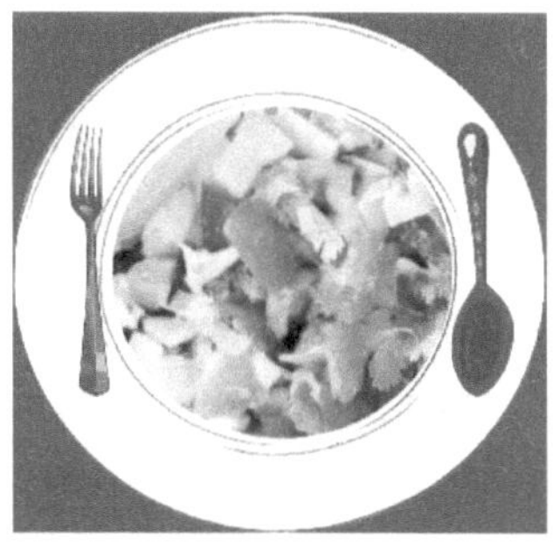

- **Serving Size:** 1 serving
- **Prep Time:** 15 minutes

Ingredients:

- 1 cup hearts of palm, sliced into thin rounds
- 1/2 cup diced tomatoes
- 1/4 cup diced red onions
- 1/4 cup diced bell peppers
- 1/4 cup chopped fresh cilantro
- Juice of 2-3 limes
- Salt and pepper to taste

Instructions:

1. In an average-sized bowl, combine together the hearts of palm, diced tomatoes, red onions, and bell peppers.
2. Drizzle the lime juice over the mixture and gently toss to combine.
3. Add the fresh cilantro, and season with salt and pepper.

4. Allow the ceviche to marinate in the refrigerator for about 15-20 minutes before serving.

Nutrient Information (per serving):

- Calories: Approximately 100-120
- Protein: 3-4 grams
- Fat: 0-1 gram
- Carbohydrates: 20-25 grams
- Fiber: 5-6 grams

Okinawan Sweet Potato Stew

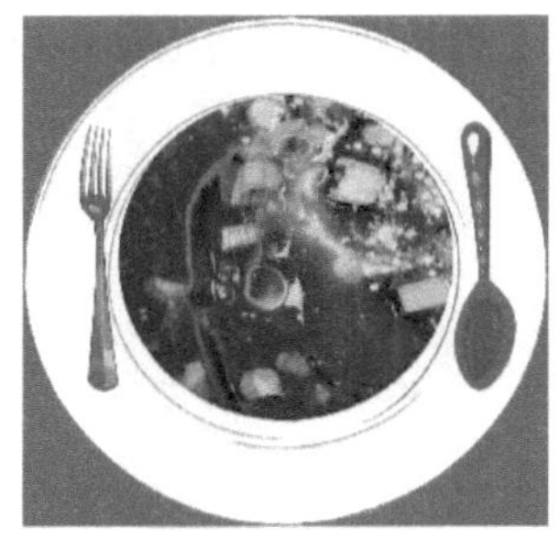

- **Serving Size:** 4 servings
- **Prep Time:** 45 minutes

Ingredients:

- 2 medium-sized Okinawan sweet potatoes, peeled and cubed
- 1 onion, chopped
- 2 cloves garlic, minced
- 2 carrots, diced
- 2 cups vegetable broth
- 1 can (14 oz) coconut milk

- 1 teaspoon curry powder
- 1/2 teaspoon turmeric
- 1/2 teaspoon cinnamon
- Salt and black pepper to taste
- Fresh cilantro for garnish (optional)

Instructions:

1. In a big-sized pot, heat some olive oil over medium heat. Add the chopped onion and garlic. Sauté until they become translucent.
2. Add the sweet potatoes, carrots, vegetable broth, and coconut milk to the pot. Season with curry powder, turmeric, cinnamon, salt, and black pepper.
3. Bring the mixture to a boil, then reduce the heat and simmer for about 30-35 minutes, or until the sweet potatoes and carrots are tender.
4. Serve the Okinawan Sweet Potato Stew hot, garnished with fresh cilantro if desired.

Pueblo Green Chile Stew

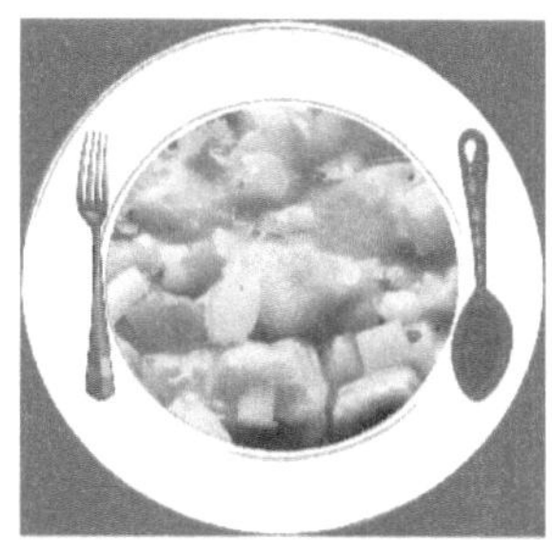

- **Serving Size:** 1 bowl
- **Prep Time:** 20 minutes + 30 minutes cooking time

Ingredients:

- 1/2 lb pork/lamb shoulder, diced
- 1/2 cup diced onion
- 1/2 cup diced green bell peppers
- 1/2 cup diced Anaheim chilies
- 1/2 cup diced tomatoes
- 1/2 cup diced potatoes
- 4 cups chicken or vegetable broth
- 2 cloves garlic, minced
- 1/2 teaspoon cumin
- Salt and black pepper to taste

Instructions:

1. In a big-sized pot, brown pork/lamb shoulder cubes.
2. Add diced onion, green bell peppers, Anaheim chilies, and minced garlic. Sauté until the vegetables are tender.
3. Stir in diced tomatoes, diced potatoes, chicken or vegetable broth, and cumin.
4. Simmer for about 20-30 minutes or until the potatoes are cooked and the flavors meld.
5. Season with salt and black pepper.

Nutrient Information (per bowl):

- Calories: Approximately 250-300
- Protein: 15-20 grams
- Fat: 10-12 grams
- Carbohydrates: 20-25 grams
- Fiber: 3-4 grams

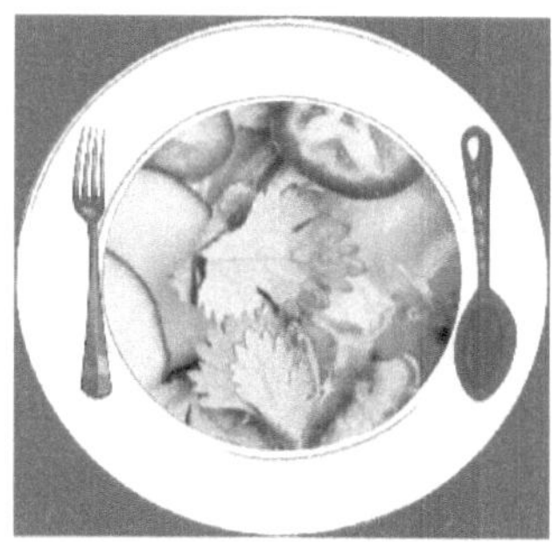

- **Serving Size:** 1 bowl
- **Prep Time:** 45 minutes

Ingredients:

- 1 cup hominy (canned or dried, prepared as per package instructions)
- 1 cup diced green tomatillos
- 1/2 cup diced green bell peppers
- 1/2 cup diced onions
- 2 cloves garlic, minced
- 1 tsp ground cumin
- 4 cups vegetable broth
- 1 cup cooked shredded chicken (optional for non-vegetarian version)
- Freshly cut cilantro, lime wedges, and shredded radishes.
- Salt and pepper to taste

Instructions:

1. In a big-sized pot, sauté the diced onions and garlic until softened.

2. Add the diced tomatillos, green bell peppers, and ground cumin, and cook until the tomatillos start to break down.
3. Add hominy and vegetable broth to the pot. Simmer and allow it to cook for approximately 20 to 25 minutes.
4. If desired, add cooked shredded chicken.
5. Season with salt and pepper.
6. Serve with garnishes like fresh cilantro, lime wedges, and sliced radishes.

Nutrient Information (per serving, without optional chicken):

- Calories: Approximately 150-180
- Protein: 4-6 grams
- Fat: 1-2 grams
- Carbohydrates: 30-35 grams
- Fiber: 5-6 grams

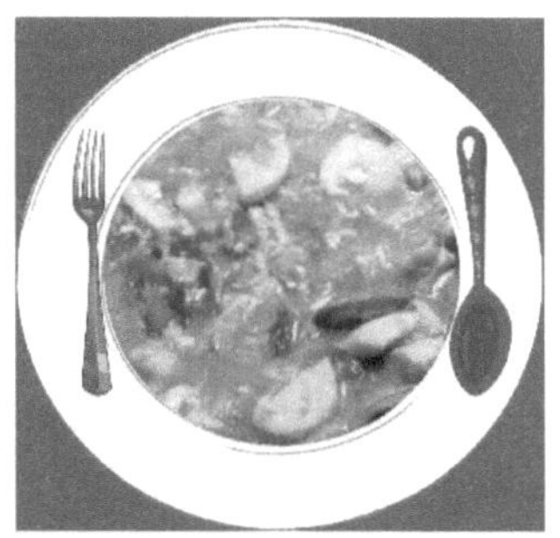

- **Serving Size:** 1 bowl
- **Prep Time:** 1 hour

Ingredients:

- 1/4 cup vegetable oil
- 1/4 cup all-purpose flour
- 1 cup diced onions
- 1/2 cup diced green bell peppers
- 1/2 cup diced celery
- 3 cloves garlic, minced
- 1 cup of frozen or fresh shredded okra
- 4 cups vegetable broth
- 1 cup diced tomatoes
- 1 cup cooked Andouille sausage (or plant-based sausage for a vegetarian version)
- 1 cup cooked shrimp (optional for non-vegetarian version)
- Cajun seasoning (to taste)
- Cooked rice for serving

Instructions:

1. In a big-sized pot, make a roux by heating vegetable oil and all-purpose flour, stirring continuously until it turns a deep brown color.
2. Add diced onions, green bell peppers, celery, and garlic to the roux, and sauté until the vegetables soften.
3. Stir in sliced okra, vegetable broth, and diced tomatoes.
4. Add Andouille sausage (or plant-based sausage) and cooked shrimp (if desired).
5. Season with Cajun seasoning to taste.
6. Simmer for about 30-40 minutes, until the gumbo thickens.
7. Serve over cooked rice.

Nutrient Information (per serving, without optional shrimp):

- Calories: Approximately 300-350
- Protein: 8-10 grams
- Fat: 15-18 grams
- Carbohydrates: 25-30 grams
- Fiber: 3-5 grams

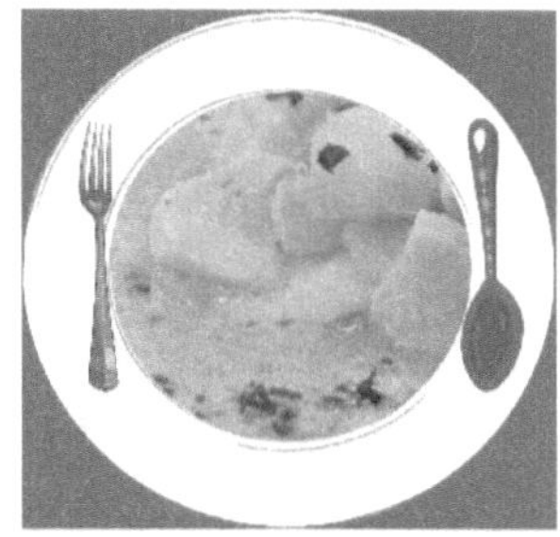

- **Serving Size:** 1 bowl
- **Prep Time:** 20 minutes + 30 minutes cooking time

Ingredients:

- 1/2 lb salmon fillet, cut into chunks
- 1/2 cup diced onion
- 1/2 cup diced celery
- 1/2 cup diced carrots
- 2 cups potatoes, peeled and diced
- 2 cups chicken or vegetable broth
- 1 cup milk
- 2 tablespoons butter
- 2 tablespoons all-purpose flour
- Salt and black pepper to taste
- Chopped fresh dill for garnish

Instructions:

1. In a big-sized pot, melt butter and sauté diced onion, celery, and carrots until they become tender.
2. Stir in diced potatoes, chicken or vegetable broth, and milk.

3. Bring the mixture to a boil and then simmer for about 15-20 minutes or until the potatoes are cooked.
4. In a separate pan, cook the salmon chunks until they are flaky.
5. In a small saucepan, create a roux by melting butter and adding all-purpose flour.
6. Gradually whisk the roux into the soup to thicken it.
7. Add cooked salmon chunks to the soup.
8. Season with salt and black pepper.
9. Garnish with chopped fresh dill before serving.

Nutrient Information (per bowl):

- Calories: Approximately 250-300
- Protein: 20-25 grams
- Fat: 10-12 grams
- Carbohydrates: 20-25 grams
- Fiber: 2-3 grams

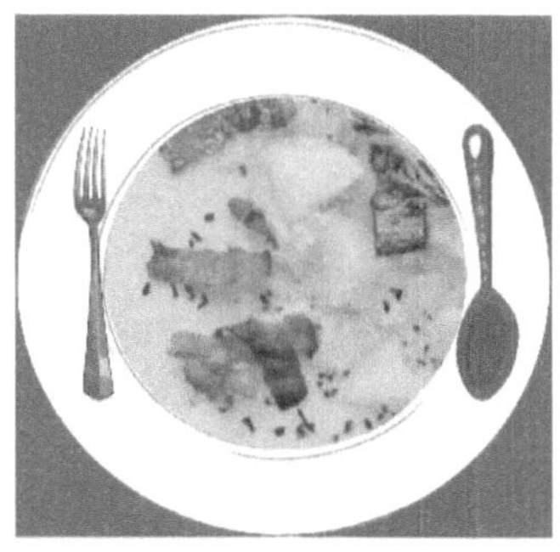

- **Serving Size:** 1 bowl
- **Prep Time:** 30 minutes

Ingredients:

- 2 slices bacon (or plant-based bacon for a vegetarian version), diced
- 1 cup diced onions
- 1/2 cup diced celery
- 1/2 cup diced carrots
- 2 cups diced potatoes
- 2 cups clam juice
- 1 cup vegetable broth
- 1 cup diced clams (canned or fresh)
- 1 cup of soy or almond milk (plant-based milk)
- 2 tbsp all-purpose flour
- Salt and pepper to taste

Instructions:

1. In a big-sized pot, cook the diced bacon (or plant-based bacon) until crispy. Take out some for garnish, while leaving the remaining in the pot.

2. Add diced onions, celery, carrots, and potatoes to the pot and sauté until the vegetables start to soften.
3. Stir in clam juice and vegetable broth, and bring to a simmer.
4. In a separate bowl, whisk together plant-based milk and all-purpose flour to create a slurry.
5. Add the slurry to the pot and continue to cook until the chowder thickens.
6. Stir in diced clams and season with salt and pepper.
7. Serve garnished with crispy bacon bits.

Nutrient Information (per serving):

- Calories: Approximately 250-300
- Protein: 10-12 grams
- Fat: 10-12 grams
- Carbohydrates: 25-30 grams
- Fiber: 3-5 grams

Clam Chowder with Milk, and Potatoes

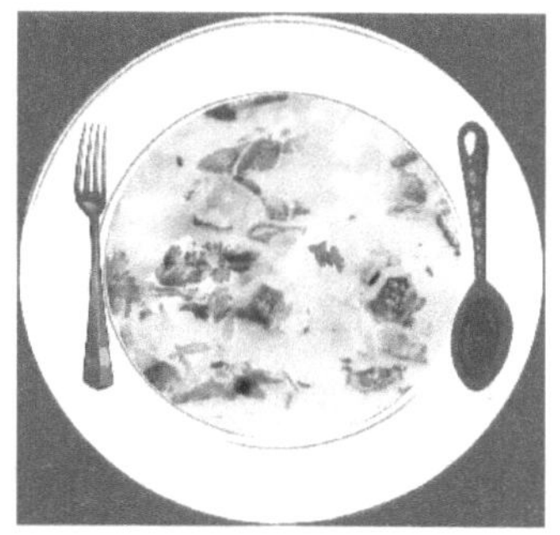

- **Serving Size:** 1 bowl
- **Prep Time:** 30 minutes

Ingredients:

- 2 cups fresh clams, cleaned and shucked (or canned clams)
- 2 cups potatoes, peeled and diced
- 1 cup milk
- 1 cup chicken or vegetable broth
- 1/2 cup diced onion
- 1/2 cup diced celery
- 2 cloves garlic, minced
- 2 tablespoons butter
- Salt and black pepper to taste
- Chopped fresh parsley for garnish

Instructions:

1. In a big-sized pot, sauté diced bacon (if using) until it becomes crispy.
2. Add diced onion and celery and sauté until they become tender.

3. Stir in minced garlic and cook for another minute.
4. Add diced potatoes, chicken or vegetable broth, and milk to the pot.
5. Simmer for about 15-20 minutes or until the potatoes are cooked.
6. Stir in shucked clams and butter, and cook until the clams are heated through.
7. Season with salt and black pepper.
8. Prior to serving, sprinkle some freshly chopped parsley on top.

Nutrient Information (per bowl):

- Calories: Approximately 250-300
- Protein: 10-15 grams
- Fat: 7-9 grams
- Carbohydrates: 30-35 grams
- Fiber: 3-4 grams

Greek Salad combined with Olives and Feta Cheese

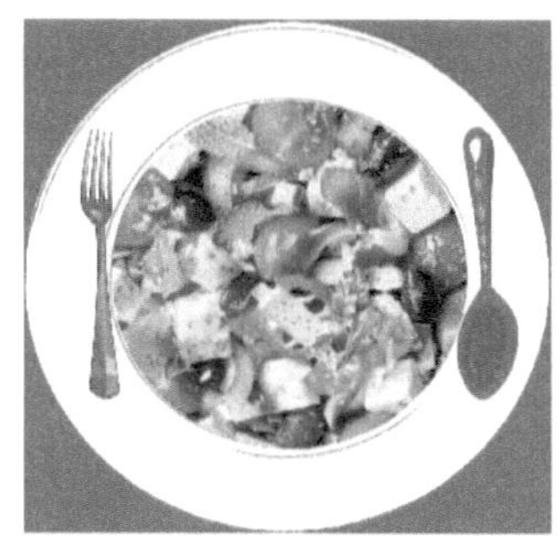

- **Serving Size**: 1 bowl (as a side)
- **Prep Time**: 15 minutes

Ingredients:

- 2 cups diced cucumbers
- 2 cups diced tomatoes
- 1/2 cup diced red onions
- 1/2 cup Kalamata olives
- 1/2 cup crumbled feta cheese
- 2 tbsp extra-virgin olive oil
- 1 tbsp red wine vinegar
- 1 tsp dried oregano
- Salt and pepper to taste

Instructions:

1. In a big-sized bowl, combine the diced cucumbers, tomatoes, red onions, and Kalamata olives.

2.   Sprinkle the crumbled feta cheese over the vegetables.

3.   Add a drizzle of red wine vinegar and super virgin olive oil.

4.   Season with dried oregano, salt, and pepper.

5.   Gently toss the ingredients to combine.

6.   Serve immediately or refrigerate for a short time to allow flavors to meld.

Nutrient Information (per serving):

- Calories: Approximately 150-200
- Protein: 5-7 grams
- Fat: 10-12 grams
- Carbohydrates: 10-15 grams
- Fiber: 3-5 grams

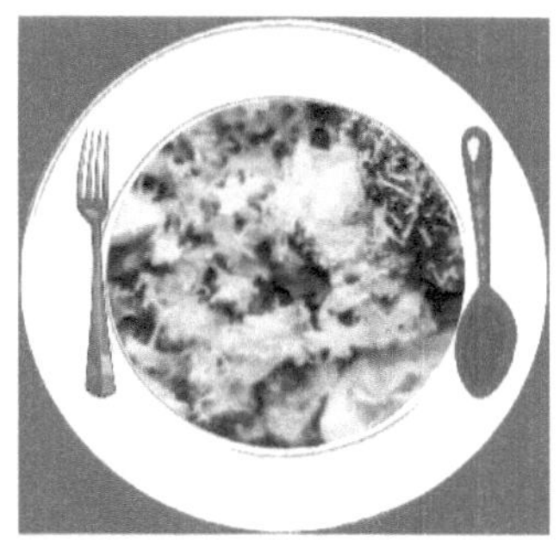

- **Serving Size:** 1 bowl (as a side)
- **Prep Time:** 20 minutes

Ingredients:

- 4 cups broccoli florets
- 2 tbsp olive oil
- Zest and juice of 1 lemon
- 1/4 cup grated Parmesan cheese
- Salt and pepper to taste

Instructions:

1. Preheat the oven to 425°F (220°C).
2. In a bowl, toss the broccoli florets with olive oil and lemon zest.
3. Spread the broccoli on a baking sheet and roast for about 15-20 minutes, or until tender and slightly crispy.
4. Drizzle the lemon juice over the roasted broccoli, sprinkle with grated Parmesan cheese, and season with salt and pepper.

Nutrient Information (per serving):

- Calories: Approximately 100-150
- Protein: 5-7 grams
- Fat: 7-9 grams
- Carbohydrates: 8-10 grams
- Fiber: 3-4 grams

Southwestern Black Bean Salad

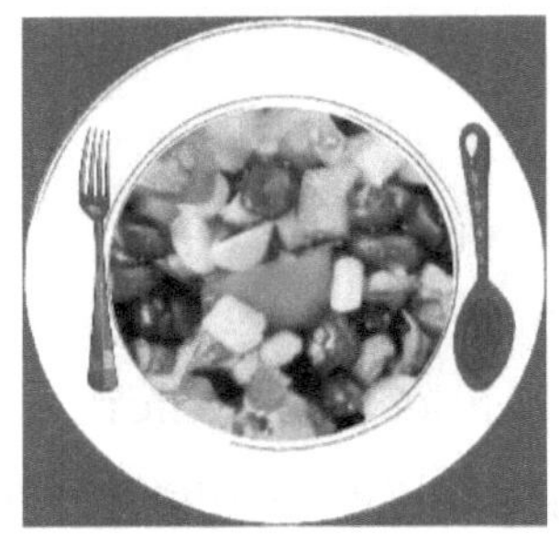

- **Serving Size:** 1 bowl (as a side)
- **Prep Time:** 20 minutes

Ingredients:

- 2 cups of black beans (canned), washed and drained
- 1 cup of thawed frozen corn kernels, or fresh
- 1 cup diced red bell peppers
- 1/2 cup diced red onions
- 1/4 cup fresh cilantro, chopped
- 1/4 cup lime juice
- 2 tbsp extra-virgin olive oil
- 1 tsp ground cumin

- Salt and pepper to taste

Instructions:

1. In an average-sized bowl, combine together the black beans, corn, diced red bell peppers, red onions, and chopped cilantro.
2. In a separate bowl, whisk together lime juice, extra-virgin olive oil, ground cumin, salt, and pepper.
3. Sprinkle the dressing on top of the salad and toss gently to combine.
4. Serve immediately or refrigerate to allow flavors to meld.

Nutrient Information (per serving):

- Calories: Approximately 150-200
- Protein: 6-8 grams
- Fat: 6-8 grams
- Carbohydrates: 20-25 grams
- Fiber: 6-8 grams

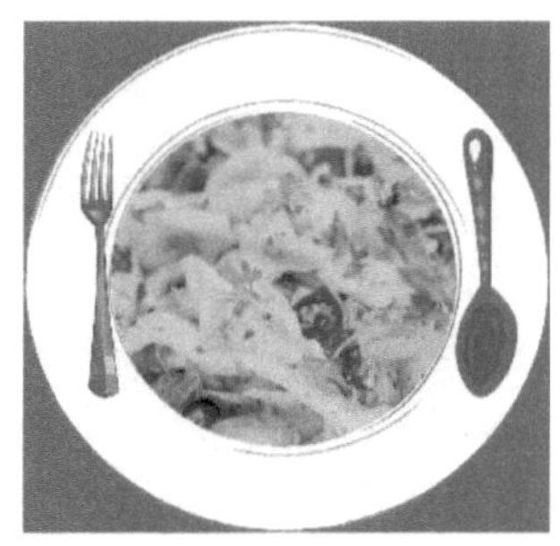

- **Serving Size:** 1 serving (as a side)
- **Prep Time:** 15 minutes

Ingredients:

- 4 cups of red and green cabbage (shredded)
- 1/2 cup shredded carrots
- 1/4 cup diced red onions
- 1/2 cup mayonnaise (or plant-based mayonnaise)
- 2 tbsp apple cider vinegar
- 1 tbsp honey. For vegan option: maple syrup
- 1 tsp Dijon mustard
- Salt and pepper to taste

Instructions:

1. In a big-sized bowl, combine the shredded cabbage, carrots, and diced red onions.
2. In a separate bowl, whisk together mayonnaise, apple cider vinegar, honey (or maple syrup), Dijon mustard, salt, and pepper.
3. Pour the dressing over the coleslaw and toss to coat.
4. Refrigerate for about 30 minutes before serving.

Nutrient Information (per serving):

- Calories: Approximately 150-200
- Protein: 1-2 grams
- Fat: 12-14 grams
- Carbohydrates:

Tuscan Kale Salad with White Beans and Lemon Vinaigrette

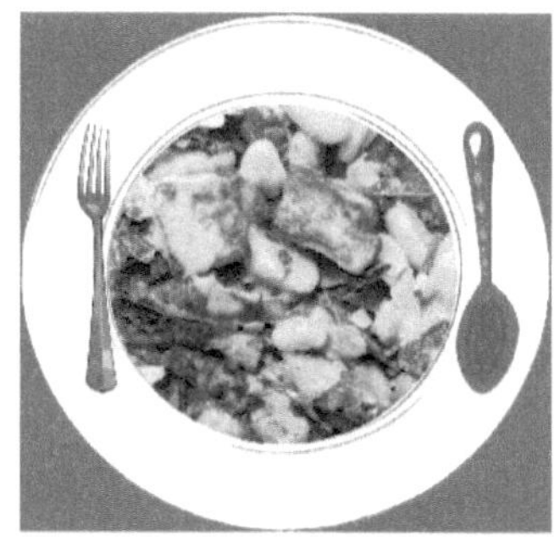

- **Serving Size:** 1 serving (as a side dish)
- **Prep Time:** 15 minutes

Ingredients:

- 2 cups Tuscan kale, washed, stemmed, and thinly sliced
- 1 cup canned white beans (e.g., cannellini beans), washed and drained
- 1/4 cup cherry tomatoes, halved
- 1/4 cup red onion, thinly sliced
- 2 tablespoons fresh lemon juice
- 2 tablespoons extra-virgin olive oil
- 1 garlic clove, minced

- 1/2 teaspoon Dijon mustard
- Salt and black pepper to taste
- Grated Parmesan cheese for garnish (optional)

Instructions:

1. In a big-sized-sized salad bowl, place the thinly sliced Tuscan kale.
2. Add the washed and drained white beans, halved cherry tomatoes, and thinly sliced red onion to the bowl with the kale.
3. In a small-sized bowl, whisk together fresh lemon juice, extra-virgin olive oil, minced garlic, Dijon mustard, salt, and black pepper to create the lemon vinaigrette.
4. Drizzle the lemon vinaigrette over the salad ingredients in the big-sized bowl.
5. Gently toss the salad to ensure that the vinaigrette is evenly distributed and coats the kale, beans, and vegetables.
6. Let the salad sit for a few minutes to allow the flavors to meld and the kale to slightly soften.
7. If desired, garnish with grated Parmesan cheese just before serving.

Nutrient Information (per serving, without Parmesan cheese):

- Calories: Approximately 200-250
- Protein: 7-9 grams
- Fat: 10-12 grams
- Carbohydrates: 20-25 grams
- Fiber: 5-7 grams

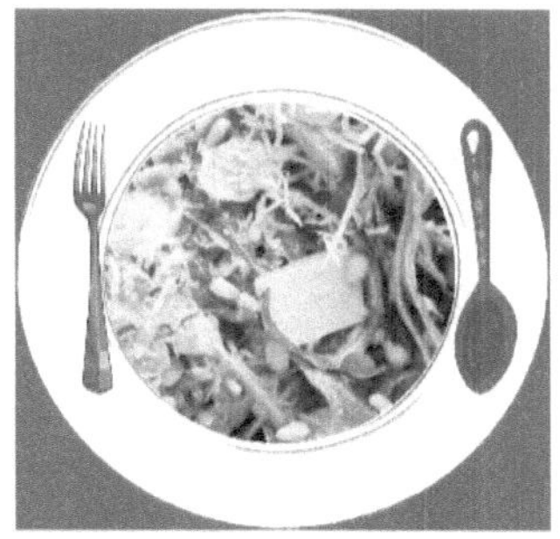

- **Serving Size:** 1 serving
- **Prep Time:** 10 minutes

Ingredients:

- 2 cups fresh arugula leaves
- 1 tablespoon lemon juice
- 1 tablespoon extra-virgin olive oil
- 1 tablespoon grated Parmesan cheese
- 1 tablespoon toasted pine nuts
- Salt and black pepper to taste

Instructions:

1. In a salad bowl, place fresh arugula leaves.
2. In a small bowl, whisk together lemon juice, extra-virgin olive oil, salt, and black pepper to create the dressing.
3. Drizzle the dressing over the arugula.
4. Sprinkle with grated Parmesan cheese and toasted pine nuts.
5.

Nutrient Information (per serving):

- Calories: Approximately 150-200
- Protein: 3-4 grams
- Fat: 12-15 grams
- Carbohydrates: 4-5 grams
- Fiber: 2-3 grams

Roasted Brussels Sprouts with Bacon and Balsamic Vinegar

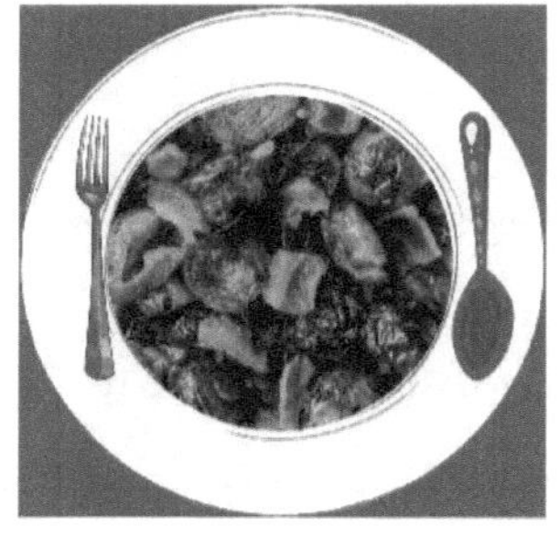

- **Serving Size:** 1 serving
- **Prep Time:** 20 minutes

Ingredients:

- 1 cup fresh Brussels sprouts, trimmed and halved
- 2 slices bacon (turkey), chopped
- 1 tablespoon balsamic vinegar
- 1 tablespoon extra-virgin olive oil
- Salt and black pepper to taste

Instructions:

1. Preheat the oven to 400°F (200°C).

2. In a bowl, toss trimmed and halved Brussels sprouts with chopped bacon, balsamic vinegar, and extra-virgin olive oil.
3. Season with salt and black pepper.
4. Spread the mixture on a baking sheet and roast for about 15-20 minutes or until the sprouts are tender and slightly crispy.

Nutrient Information (per serving):

- Calories: Approximately 200-250
- Protein: 6-8 grams
- Fat: 15-20 grams
- Carbohydrates: 7-9 grams
- Fiber: 3-4 grams

Mashed Sweet Potatoes with Marshmallows and Cinnamon

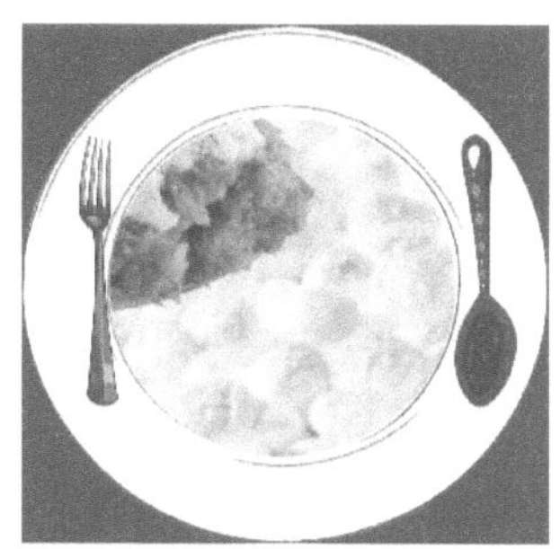

- **Serving Size:** 1 serving
- **Prep Time:** 30 minutes

Ingredients:

- 1 cup mashed sweet potatoes

- 1/4 cup mini marshmallows
- 1/2 teaspoon ground cinnamon

Instructions:

1. Preheat the oven to 350°F (175°C).
2. In a baking dish, spread the mashed sweet potatoes.
3. Sprinkle mini marshmallows over the top.
4. Dust with ground cinnamon.
5. Bake for about 15-20 minutes or until the marshmallows are toasted and the dish is heated through.

Nutrient Information (per serving):

- Calories: Approximately 200-250
- Protein: 2-3 grams
- Fat: 0-1 gram
- Carbohydrates: 45-50 grams
- Fiber: 3-4 grams

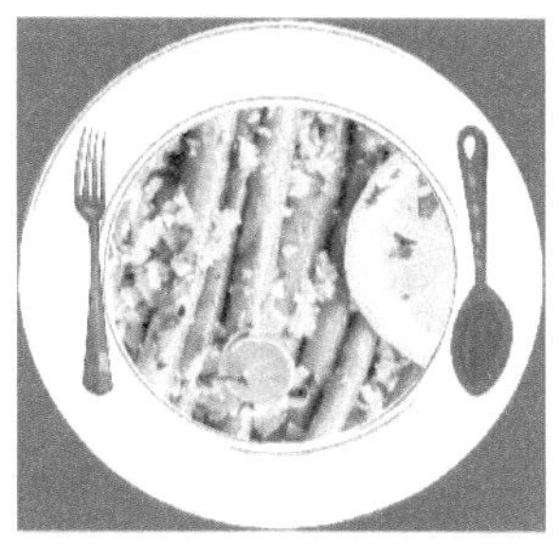

- **Serving Size:** 1 serving
- **Prep Time:** 10 minutes

Ingredients:

- 1 cup fresh asparagus spears, trimmed
- 1/2 lemon, juiced
- 1 tablespoon melted butter
- Salt and black pepper to taste

Instructions:

1. Warm up a grill or grill pan to a temperature of about medium-high.
2. Toss trimmed asparagus spears with melted butter and season with salt and black pepper.
3. Grill the asparagus for about 5-7 minutes or until they are tender and slightly charred.
4. Squeeze fresh lemon juice over the grilled asparagus before serving.

Nutrient Information (per serving):

- Calories: Approximately 100-150
- Protein: 2-3 grams

- Fat: 9-10 grams
- Carbohydrates: 4-5 grams
- Fiber: 2-3 grams

Roasted Cauliflower with Parmesan Cheese

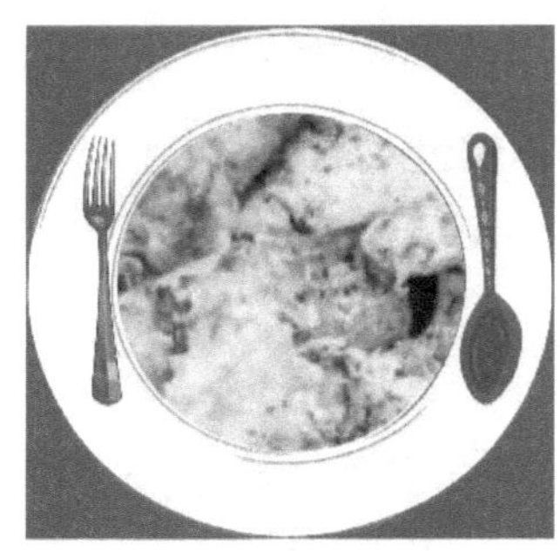

- **Serving Size:** 1 serving
- **Prep Time:** 20 minutes

Ingredients:

- 1 cup cauliflower florets
- 1 tablespoon olive oil
- 1/4 cup grated Parmesan cheese
- 1/2 teaspoon garlic powder
- Salt and black pepper to taste

Instructions:

1. Preheat the oven to 425°F (220°C).
2. In a bowl, toss cauliflower florets with olive oil, grated Parmesan cheese, garlic powder, salt, and black pepper.

3. Spread the cauliflower on a baking sheet and roast for about 20-25 minutes or until it's tender and golden brown.

Nutrient Information (per serving):

- Calories: Approximately 150-200
- Protein: 6-8 grams
- Fat: 10-12 grams
- Carbohydrates: 7-9 grams
- Fiber: 3-4 grams

MAIN COURSES

Southwestern Quinoa Burgers

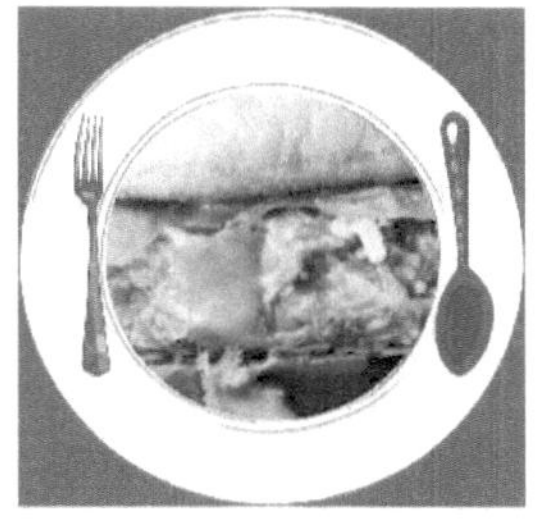

- **Serving Size:** 1 quinoa burger
- **Prep Time:** 30 minutes

Ingredients:

- 1 cup cooked quinoa
- 1 15 oz tin of black beans, washed and drained
- 1/2 cup of thawed frozen corn kernels, or fresh
- 1/4 cup diced red onions

- 1/4 cup diced red bell peppers
- 2 cloves garlic, minced
- 1 tsp ground cumin
- 1 tsp chili powder
- Salt and pepper to taste
- 1/4 cup breadcrumbs (whole-grain for a healthier option)
- 1/4 cup chopped fresh cilantro
- Cooking spray or olive oil for pan-frying
- Whole-grain burger buns
- Choose toppings that you prefer such as avocado, lettuce, tomato, etc.)

Instructions:

1. In a big-sized bowl, combine cooked quinoa, black beans, corn, red onions, red bell peppers, garlic, ground cumin, chili powder, salt, and pepper.
2. Add breadcrumbs and chopped cilantro, and mix until the mixture holds together.
3. Form the mixture into burger patties.
4. Heat up the pan over moderate-high flame, lightly spray with cooking spray or olive oil, and cook the quinoa burgers for about 4-5 minutes per side, until they're golden brown and heated through.
5. Serve the quinoa burgers on whole-grain buns with your choice of toppings.

Nutrient Information (per quinoa burger, without bun and toppings):

- Calories: Approximately 150-200

- Protein: 6-8 grams
- Fat: 2-4 grams
- Carbohydrates: 30-35 grams
- Fiber: 6-8 grams

Vegetarian Chili Mac

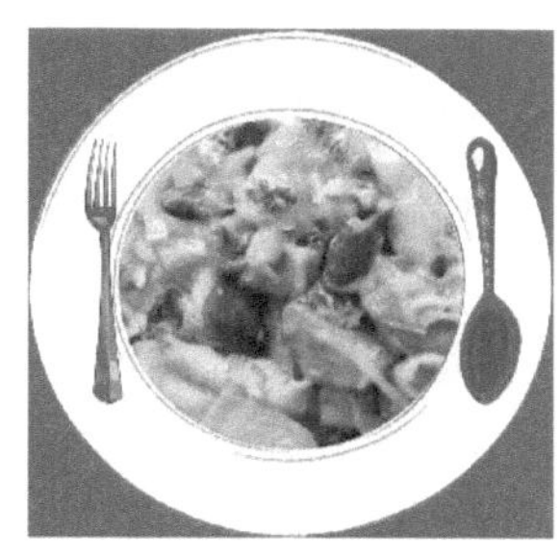

- **Serving Size:** 1 bowl
- **Prep Time:** 30 minutes

Ingredients:

- 1 cup whole-grain macaroni or pasta of your choice
- 1 15 oz tin of black beans, washed and drained
- 1 cup diced tomatoes
- 1/2 cup of thawed frozen corn kernels, or fresh
- 1/2 cup diced red bell peppers
- 1/4 cup diced red onions
- 2 cloves garlic, minced
- 1 tsp chili powder
- 1/2 tsp ground cumin
- Salt and pepper to taste
- For garnish: lime wedges or fresh cilantro

Instructions:

1. Cook the whole-grain macaroni or pasta according to the package instructions and set aside.
2. In a big-sized skillet, combine black beans, diced tomatoes, corn, red bell peppers, red onions, garlic, chili powder, ground cumin, salt, and pepper.
3. Simmer the mixture for about 10 minutes until heated through and the flavors meld.
4. Serve the chili mixture over cooked pasta, garnished with fresh cilantro and lime wedges.

Nutrient Information (per serving):

- Calories: Approximately 350-400
- Protein: 12-15 grams
- Fat: 2-4 grams
- Carbohydrates: 70-75 grams
- Fiber: 12-15 grams

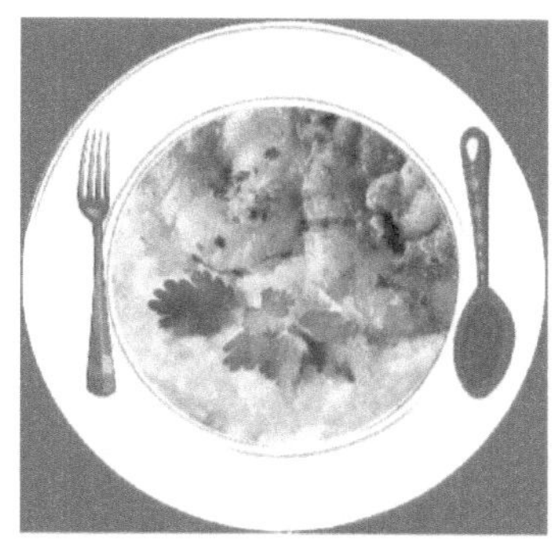

- **Serving Size:** 1 serving
- **Prep Time:** 30 minutes

Ingredients:

- 1/2 cup stone-ground grits
- 1 cup water
- 1 cup low-sodium chicken broth
- 1/2 lb fresh shrimp that has been deveined and peeled
- 1/4 cup diced onions
- 1/4 cup diced green bell peppers
- 2 cloves garlic, minced
- 1/2 cup diced tomatoes
- 2 tbsp diced scallions
- 2 tbsp chopped fresh parsley
- 1/4 cup chicken broth
- 1/4 tsp Old Bay seasoning
- Salt and pepper to taste
- 1 tsp olive oil

Instructions:

1. In a saucepan, combine water and low-sodium chicken broth, and bring to a boil.
2. Stir in stone-ground grits, reduce heat to low, and simmer, stirring occasionally, for about 20-25 minutes until the grits are creamy and tender.
3. Season the shrimp with Old Bay seasoning, salt, and pepper.
4. In a skillet, heat olive oil over medium heat, and sauté diced onions, green bell peppers, and garlic until softened.
5. Add the diced tomatoes and shrimp, and cook until the shrimp are pink and cooked through.
6. Stir in diced scallions, chopped fresh parsley, and chicken broth.
7. Serve the shrimp and vegetable mixture over a serving of creamy grits.

Nutrient Information (per serving):

- Calories: Approximately 300-350
- Protein: 20-25 grams
- Fat: 6-8 grams
- Carbohydrates: 40-45 grams
- Fiber: 3-5 grams

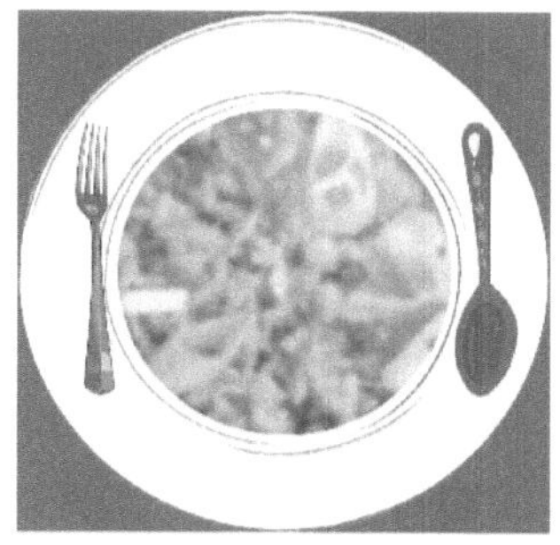

- **Serving Size:** 1 bowl
- **Prep Time:** 20 minutes + 45 minutes cooking time

Ingredients:

- 1/2 cup okra, sliced
- 1/2 cup bell peppers, chopped
- 1/2 cup celery, chopped
- 1/2 cup onion, chopped
- 1/2 cup tomatoes, chopped
- 1/2 cup cooked shrimp
- 1/2 cup cooked chicken, shredded
- 1/2 cup cooked sausage, sliced
- 4 cups chicken broth
- 1/4 cup roux (a mixture of flour and oil)
- 1/2 teaspoon cayenne pepper
- 1/2 teaspoon black pepper
- Salt to taste
- Cooked rice for serving

Instructions:

1. In a big-sized pot, heat the roux over medium heat until it becomes brown (like a caramel color), stirring constantly to avoid burning.
2. Add the chopped okra, bell peppers, celery, and onions to the roux, and continue to cook for about 10 minutes.
3. Stir in the chopped tomatoes, chicken broth, cayenne pepper, black pepper, and salt.
4. Simmer for about 20-30 minutes.
5. Add the cooked shrimp, chicken, and sausage to the gumbo and cook until heated through.
6. Serve over cooked rice.

Nutrient Information (per bowl, without rice):

- Calories: Approximately 300-350
- Protein: 20-25 grams
- Fat: 15-20 grams
- Carbohydrates: 20-25 grams
- Fiber: 3-5 grams

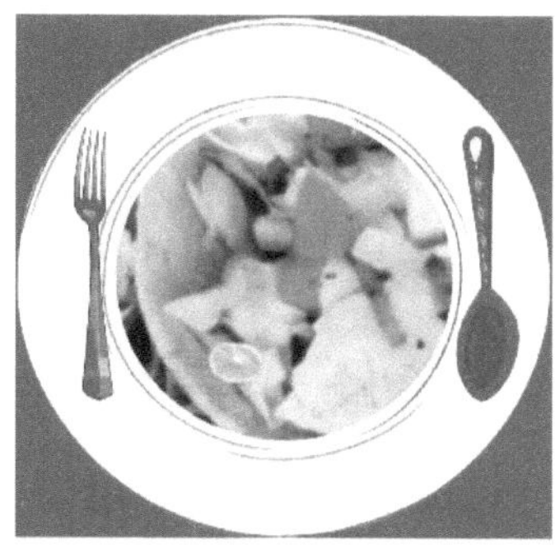

- **Serving Size:** 1 taco
- **Prep Time:** 20 minutes

Ingredients:

- 1 white fish fillet (e.g., cod, tilapia)
- 1/2 cup shredded lettuce
- 1/4 cup diced tomatoes
- 1/4 cup diced red onion
- 2 tablespoons chopped cilantro
- 1 lime, cut into wedges
- 2 small corn tortillas
- 1 tablespoon plain Greek yogurt
- 1/2 teaspoon hot sauce (optional)
- Salt and black pepper to taste

Instructions:

1. Season the white fish fillet with salt and black pepper.
2. Grill or pan-fry the fish until it's cooked through.
3. In a small-sized bowl, mix plain Greek yogurt and hot sauce (if using) to create a creamy sauce.

4. Heat the corn tortillas until warm and pliable.

5. Assemble the tacos by placing shredded lettuce, diced tomatoes, diced red onion, and chopped cilantro on each tortilla.

6. Top with grilled fish and a drizzle of the creamy sauce.

7. Serve with lime wedges.

Nutrient Information (per taco):

- Calories: Approximately 150-200
- Protein: 15-20 grams
- Fat: 2-3 grams
- Carbohydrates: 15-20 grams
- Fiber: 3-4 grams

Cajun Blackened Salmon

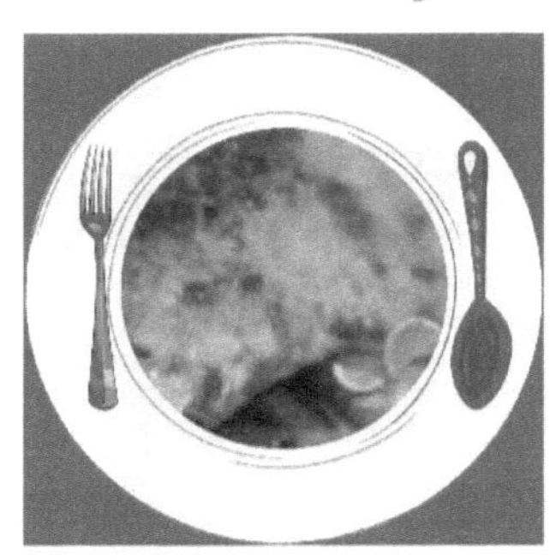

- **Serving Size:** 1 salmon fillet
- **Prep Time:** 20 minutes

Ingredients:

- 1 salmon fillet (6-8 oz)

- 1 tbsp of homemade or store-bought Cajun seasoning
- 1 tsp olive oil
- Lemon wedges for serving

Instructions:

1. Preheat a cast-iron skillet over high heat until it's very hot.
2. Rub both sides of the salmon fillet with Cajun seasoning.
3. Drizzle olive oil over the fillet.
4. Place the salmon in the hot skillet and cook for about 2-3 minutes on each side, until it's blackened and cooked to your desired level of doneness.
5. Serve with lemon wedges.

Nutrient Information (per salmon fillet, without lemon wedges):

- Calories: Approximately 300-350
- Protein: 20-25 grams
- Fat: 15-20 grams
- Carbohydrates: 2-4 grams
- Fiber: 1-2 grams

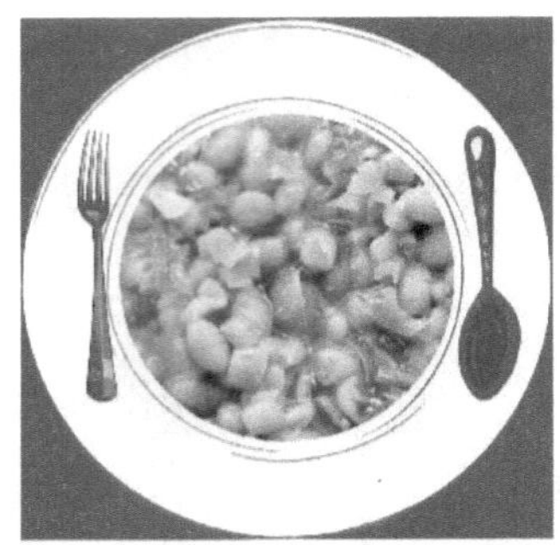

- **Serving Size:** 1 cup
- **Prep Time:** 10 minutes (plus soaking time) + 2 hours cooking time

Ingredients:

- 1 cup dried navy beans
- 1/2 cup molasses
- 1/4 cup brown sugar
- 1/4 cup ketchup
- 1 onion, diced
- 1 teaspoon dry mustard
- 1/4 teaspoon black pepper
- 1/4 teaspoon salt
- 1/4 teaspoon ground cloves
- 4 cups water

Instructions:

1. Soak the dried navy beans in water overnight or for at least 8 hours.
2. Preheat your oven to 325°F (165°C).

3. In a baking dish, combine the soaked beans, molasses, brown sugar, ketchup, diced onion, dry mustard, black pepper, salt, and ground cloves.

4. Pour enough water such that it will cover up the beans.

5. Cover the dish and bake for about 2 hours or until the beans are tender. If more water is required while baking, add it.

6. Uncover the dish during the last 30 minutes of baking to thicken the sauce.

Nutrient Information (per cup):

- Calories: Approximately 200-250
- Protein: 7-9 grams
- Fat: 1-2 grams
- Carbohydrates: 45-50 grams
- Fiber: 7-9 grams

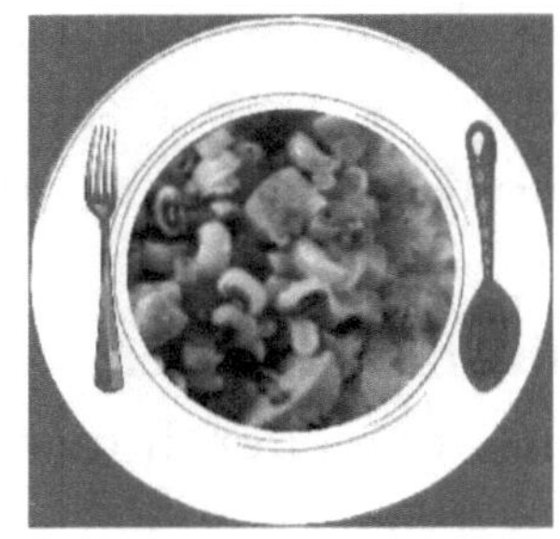

- **Serving Size:** 1 cup
- **Prep Time:** 15 minutes + 45 minutes cooking time

Ingredients:

- 1 cup of cooked or canned black-eyed peas
- 1 cup long-grain white rice
- 1 onion, chopped
- 1 green bell pepper, chopped
- 2 cloves garlic, minced
- 2 cups chicken or vegetable broth
- 1/2 teaspoon black pepper
- 1/4 teaspoon cayenne pepper
- Salt to taste
- Sliced green onions for garnish

Instructions:

1. In a big-sized pot, sauté chopped onions and green bell peppers until they become tender.
2. Add minced garlic and continue to sauté for another minute.

3. Stir in cooked or canned black-eyed peas, long-grain white rice, chicken or vegetable broth, black pepper, cayenne pepper, and salt.
4. Bring the mixture to a boil, then reduce the heat, cover, and simmer for about 20-25 minutes or until the rice is cooked and the liquid is absorbed.
5. Garnish with sliced green onions before serving.

Nutrient Information (per cup):

- Calories: Approximately 200-250
- Protein: 7-9 grams
- Fat: 1-2 grams
- Carbohydrates: 40-45 grams
- Fiber: 5-7 grams

Salmon with Roasted Vegetables and Lemon Aioli

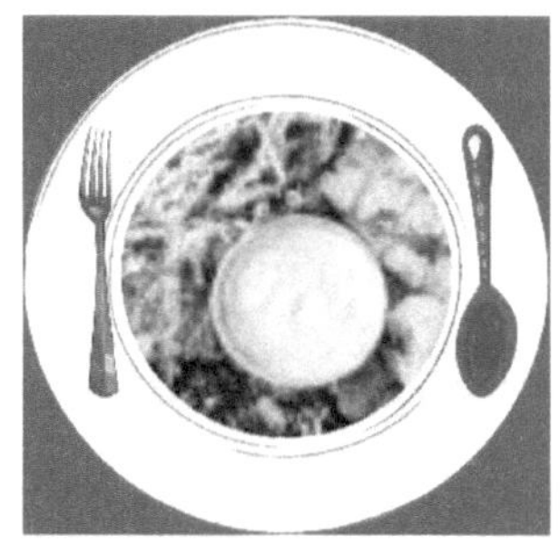

- Serving Size: 1 serving
- Prep Time: 30 minutes

Ingredients:

- 1 salmon fillet

- 1 cup mixed roasted vegetables (e.g., carrots, zucchini, bell peppers)
- 1 tablespoon olive oil
- 1/2 lemon, juiced
- 2 tablespoons mayonnaise
- 1/2 garlic clove, minced
- Salt and black pepper to taste

Instructions:

1. Preheat the oven to 375°F (190°C).
2. Toss mixed roasted vegetables with olive oil, salt, and black pepper.
3. Roast in the oven for about 20-25 minutes or until they are tender and slightly caramelized.
4. Season the salmon fillet with olive oil, lemon juice, salt, and black pepper. Grill or bake until the salmon is cooked through.
5. In a small bowl, mix mayonnaise, minced garlic, and a squeeze of lemon juice to create the lemon aioli.
6. Serve the salmon with the roasted vegetables and a drizzle of lemon aioli.

Nutrient Information (per serving):

- Calories: Approximately 300-350
- Protein: 20-25 grams
- Fat: 20-25 grams
- Carbohydrates: 15-20 grams
- Fiber: 3-4 grams

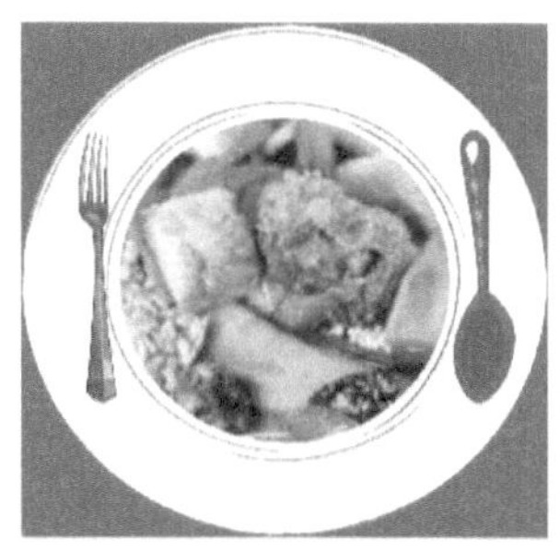

- **Serving Size:** 1 serving
- **Prep Time:** 30 minutes

Ingredients:

- 4 oz tofu, cubed
- 1 cup mixed vegetables (e.g., broccoli, bell peppers, snap peas)
- 1/2 cup cooked brown rice
- 1 tablespoon low-sodium soy sauce
- 1/2 teaspoon ginger, minced
- 1/2 teaspoon garlic, minced
- 1/2 teaspoon sesame oil
- 1/2 teaspoon honey or maple syrup (optional)
- 1/2 teaspoon cornstarch (optional)
- Sesame seeds for garnish (optional)

Instructions:

1. In a bowl, marinate tofu cubes with low-sodium soy sauce, ginger, garlic, and sesame oil.
2. Heat a skillet or wok over high heat and stir-fry the tofu until it's browned and cooked through.
3. Remove the tofu from the skillet.

4. In the same skillet, stir-fry mixed vegetables until they are tender-crisp.
5. Add the cooked brown rice to the skillet and stir-fry to heat through.
6. If desired, mix cornstarch with a little water and stir into the stir-fry to create a thicker sauce.
7. Serve the tofu stir-fry with a drizzle of honey or maple syrup (if desired) and garnish with sesame seeds.

Nutrient Information (per serving, without optional ingredients):

- Calories: Approximately 300-350
- Protein: 15-20 grams
- Fat: 10-12 grams
- Carbohydrates: 40-45 grams
- Fiber: 5-7 grams

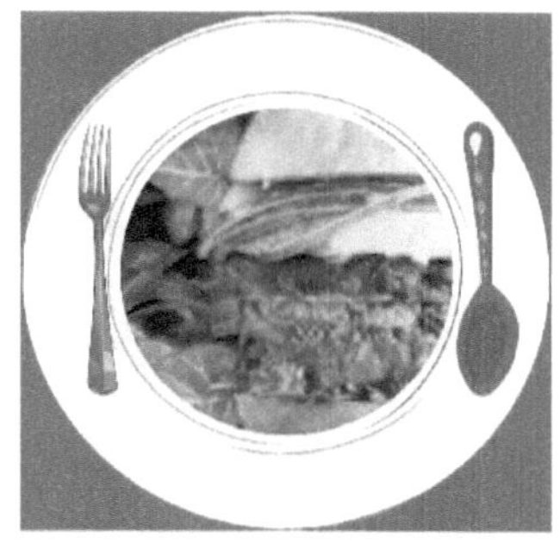

- **Serving Size**: 1 burger with fries
- Prep Time: 45 minutes

Ingredients:

For the lentil burgers:

- 1 cup cooked lentils
- 1/2 cup bread crumbs
- 1/4 cup finely chopped onion
- 1/4 cup finely chopped bell pepper
- 1/4 cup grated carrot
- 1/4 cup chopped parsley
- 1 teaspoon garlic powder
- 1/2 teaspoon cumin
- Salt and black pepper to taste

For the sweet potato fries:

- 1 sweet potato, cut into fries
- 1 tablespoon olive oil
- 1/2 teaspoon paprika
- 1/4 teaspoon garlic powder

- Salt and black pepper to taste
- Whole-wheat burger buns and toppings of your choice (lettuce, tomato, onion, etc.)

Instructions: For the lentil burgers:

1. In a bowl, mash cooked lentils.
2. Add bread crumbs, chopped onion, bell pepper, grated carrot, parsley, garlic powder, cumin, salt, and black pepper. Mix until well combined.
3. Shape the mixture into burger patties.
4. Heat a skillet and cook the lentil burgers until they are browned and heated through.

For the sweet potato fries:

1. Preheat the oven to 425°F (220°C).
2. Toss sweet potato fries with olive oil, paprika, garlic powder, salt, and black pepper.
3. Spread the fries on a baking sheet and bake for about 20-25 minutes or until they are crispy and browned.

Assemble the lentil burgers on whole-wheat buns with your choice of toppings and serve with sweet potato fries.

Nutrient Information (per burger with fries):

- Calories: Approximately 350-400 (burger) + 100-150 (fries)
- Protein: 15-20 grams (burger) + 2-3 grams (fries)
- Fat: 5-7 grams (burger) + 4-6 grams (fries)
- Carbohydrates: 60-70 grams (burger) + 20-25 grams (fries)
- Fiber: 10-12 grams (burger) + 3-4 grams (fries)

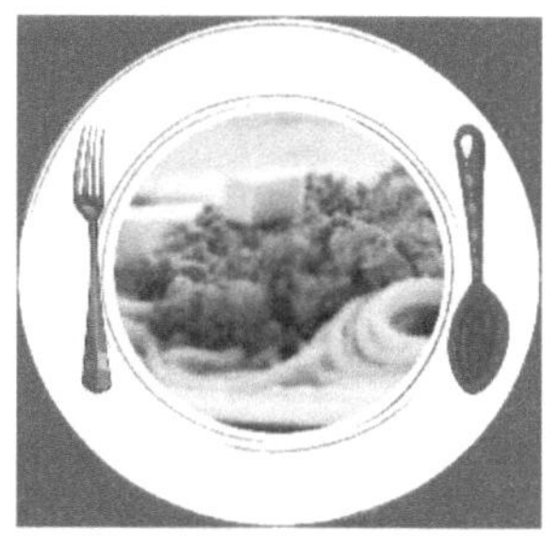

- Serving Size: 1 serving
- Prep Time: 30 minutes

Ingredients:

- 2 oz whole-wheat spaghetti
- 1/2 cup lentils, cooked
- 1/2 cup diced tomatoes
- 1/4 cup diced onion
- 1/4 cup diced bell pepper
- 1/4 cup grated carrot
- 1/4 cup sliced mushrooms
- 1 teaspoon garlic, minced
- 1/2 teaspoon dried oregano
- 1/2 teaspoon dried basil
- Salt and black pepper to taste
- Grated Parmesan cheese for garnish (optional)

Instructions:

1. Cook the whole-wheat spaghetti in accordance to instructions that was given on the package.

2. In a skillet, sauté diced onion, bell pepper, grated carrot, sliced mushrooms, and minced garlic until they become tender.
3. Add cooked lentils, diced tomatoes, dried oregano, dried basil, salt, and black pepper. Simmer to combine and heat through.
4. Serve the vegetarian Bolognese sauce over cooked whole-wheat spaghetti.
5. If preferred, sprinkle some grated Parmesan cheese on top.

Nutrient Information (per serving, without optional ingredients):

- Calories: Approximately 250-300
- Protein: 12-15 grams
- Fat: 1-2 grams
- Carbohydrates: 50-55 grams
- Fiber: 10-12 grams

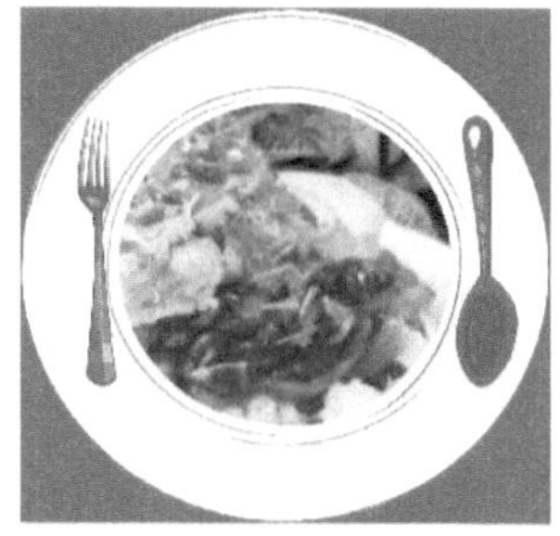

- Serving Size: 1 serving
- Prep Time: 30 minutes

Ingredients:

- 4 oz sliced chicken breast, devoid bone and skin
- 1/2 cup sliced bell peppers
- 1/2 cup sliced onion
- 1/2 cup cooked brown rice
- 1/2 cup cooked black beans
- 1 tablespoon olive oil
- 1/2 teaspoon chili powder
- 1/2 teaspoon cumin
- 1/2 teaspoon paprika
- Salt and black pepper to taste
- Fresh cilantro for garnish (optional)

Instructions:

1. Preheat the oven to 400°F (200°C).
2. In a bowl, combine chicken slices, sliced bell peppers, sliced onion, olive oil, chili powder, cumin, paprika, salt, and black pepper.

3. Spread the mixture on a baking sheet and roast for about 20-25 minutes or until the chicken is cooked through and the vegetables are tender.
4. Serve the chicken fajitas with cooked brown rice and black beans.
5. If preferred, sprinkle some fresh cilantro on top.

Nutrient Information (per serving):

- Calories: Approximately 350-400
- Protein: 25-30 grams
- Fat: 7-9 grams
- Carbohydrates: 40-45 grams
- Fiber: 8-10 grams

Key Lime Pie

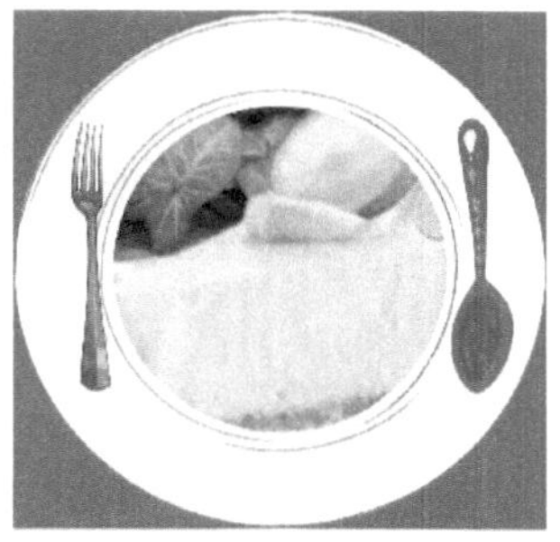

- **Serving Size:** 1 slice
- **Prep Time:** 20 minutes (and the time for chilling)

Ingredients:

For the crust:

- 1 1/2 cups graham cracker crumbs
- 1/4 cup granulated sugar
- 1/2 cup melted unsalted butter (or plant-based butter)

For the filling:

- 1 can (14 oz) sweetened condensed milk (or a dairy-free alternative)
- 4 big-sized egg yolks (or egg substitutes if desired)
- 1/2 cup fresh key lime juice (or regular lime juice)
- 1 tbsp lime zest

Optional topping: whipped cream or whipped coconut cream

Instructions:

1. Preheat the oven to 350°F (175°C).
2. In an average-sized bowl, combine together graham cracker crumbs, granulated sugar, and melted butter.
3. Press the mixture into a pie dish to form the crust.
4. In a separate bowl, whisk together sweetened condensed milk, egg yolks, key lime juice, and lime zest.
5. Pour the filling into the crust.
6. Bake for about 15-20 minutes until the filling is set.
7. Allow the pie to cool, then refrigerate for a few hours or until well-chilled.
8. Serve with a dollop of whipped cream or whipped coconut cream if desired.

Nutrient Information (per slice, without topping):

- Calories: Approximately 250-300
- Protein: 5-7 grams
- Fat: 12-15 grams
- Carbohydrates: 30-35 grams
- Fiber: 1-2 grams

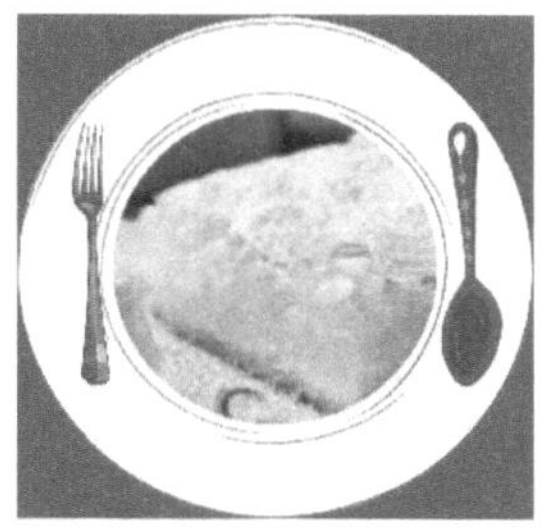

- **Serving Size:** 1 bar
- **Prep Time:** 40 minutes

Ingredients:

For the crust:

- 1 cup all-purpose flour
- 1/2 cup of softened butter that is unsalted (or plant-based butter)
- 1/4 cup powdered sugar

For the lemon topping:

- 2 big-sized eggs (or egg substitutes if desired)
- 1 cup granulated sugar
- 2 tbsp all-purpose flour
- 1/4 cup lemon juice
- 1 tsp lemon zest
- 1/2 tsp baking powder

Powdered sugar for dusting

Instructions:

1. Preheat the oven to 350°F (175°C).

2. In an average-sized bowl, combine together all-purpose flour, softened butter, and powdered sugar to form the crust mixture.

3. Press the crust mixture into the bottom of a baking pan.

4. Bake the crust for about 15-20 minutes until lightly golden.

5. In another bowl, whisk together eggs, granulated sugar, all-purpose flour, lemon juice, lemon zest, and baking powder.

6. Cover the cooked crust with the lemon topping.

7. Bake for an additional 20-25 minutes or until the topping is set.

8. Allow the bars to cool, then dust with powdered sugar before cutting into bars.

Nutrient Information (per bar, with powdered sugar dusting):

- Calories: Approximately 150-200
- Protein: 2-4 grams
- Fat: 8-10 grams
- Carbohydrates: 20-25 grams
- Fiber: 1-2 grams

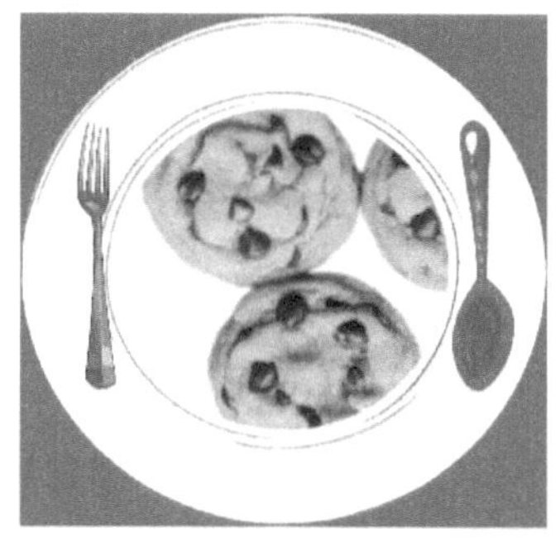

- **Serving Size:** 1 cookie
- **Prep Time:** 30 minutes

Ingredients:

- 1/2 cup of softened butter that is unsalted (or plant-based butter)
- 1/2 cup granulated sugar
- 1/4 cup brown sugar
- 1 big-sized egg (or egg substitute)
- 1 tsp pure vanilla extract
- 1 1/4 cups all-purpose flour
- 1/2 tsp baking soda
- 1/2 tsp salt
- 1 cup semisweet chocolate chips

Instructions:

1. Preheat the oven to 350°F (175°C).
2. In a bowl, cream together softened butter, granulated sugar, and brown sugar until smooth.
3. Include the egg and vanilla extract and beat until it is well combined.

4. In a different bowl, put together all-purpose flour, salt, and baking soda.

5. Gradually add the dry ingredients to the wet ingredients and mix until just incorporated.

6. Fold in the semisweet chocolate chips.

7. Drop dough by rounded tablespoons onto ungreased baking sheets.

8. Bake for 10-12 minutes until the cookies are lightly golden around the edges.

9. Allow them to cool on the baking sheets for a few minutes before transferring to a wire rack to cool completely.

Nutrient Information (per cookie):

- Calories: Approximately 100-150
- Protein: 1-2 grams
- Fat: 5-7 grams
- Carbohydrates: 15-20 grams
- Fiber: 1-2 grams

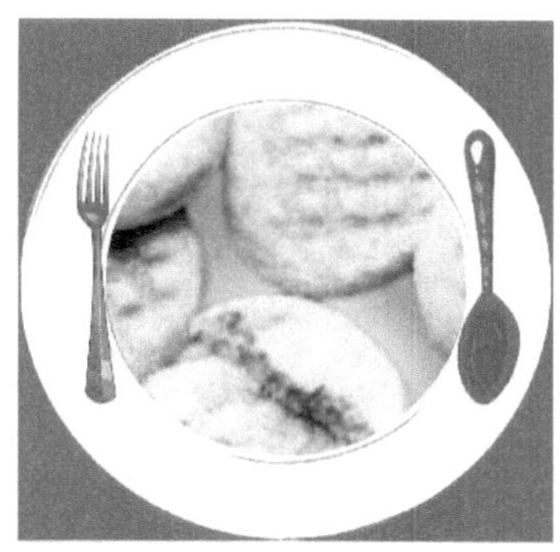

- **Serving Size:** 1 cookie
- **Prep Time:** 30 minutes

Ingredients:

- 1/2 cup of softened butter that is unsalted (or plant-based butter)
- 1/2 cup peanut butter
- 1/2 cup granulated sugar
- 1/2 cup brown sugar
- 1 big-sized egg (or egg substitute)
- 1 tsp pure vanilla extract
- 1 1/4 cups all-purpose flour
- 1/2 tsp baking powder
- 1/2 tsp baking soda
- 1/4 tsp salt

Instructions:

1. Preheat the oven to 350°F (175°C).
2. In a bowl, cream together softened butter, peanut butter, granulated sugar, and brown sugar until smooth.

3. Include the egg and vanilla extract and beat until it is well combined.
4. In a different bowl, put together all-purpose flour, baking powder, baking soda, and salt.
5. Gradually add the dry ingredients to the wet ingredients and mix until just incorporated.
6. Shape the dough into 1-inch balls and place them on ungreased baking sheets.
7. On each cookie, make a crosshatch design with a fork.
8. Bake for 10-12 minutes until the cookies are lightly golden.
9. Allow them to cool on the baking sheets for a few minutes before transferring to a wire rack to cool completely.

Nutrient Information (per cookie):

- Calories: Approximately 100-150
- Protein: 2-3 grams
- Fat: 6-8 grams
- Carbohydrates: 10-15 grams
- Fiber: 1-2 grams

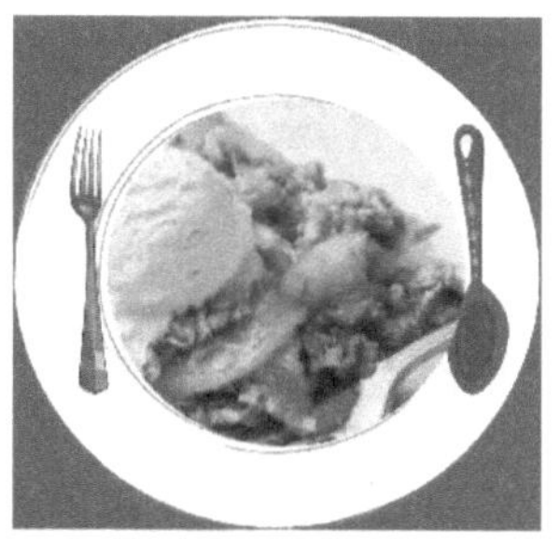

- **Serving Size:** 1 serving
- **Prep Time:** 45 minutes

Ingredients:

For the apple filling:

- 4 cups of already peeled and sliced such as Granny Smith
- 2 tbsp granulated sugar
- 1/2 tsp ground cinnamon
- 1/4 tsp ground nutmeg

For the crisp topping:

- 1/2 cup rolled oats
- 1/4 cup all-purpose flour
- 1/4 cup brown sugar
- 1/4 cup unsalted butter (or plant-based butter), softened

Serve with yogurt or vanilla ice cream (optional).

Instructions:

1. Preheat the oven to 350°F (175°C).

2. In an average-sized bowl, combine together sliced and peeled apples with granulated sugar, ground cinnamon, and ground nutmeg.
3. Transfer the apple mixture to a baking dish.
4. In another bowl, mix rolled oats, all-purpose flour, brown sugar, and softened butter to create the crisp topping.
5. On the apples, spread the crisp topping.
6. Bake for about 30-35 minutes until the topping is golden brown and the apples are tender.
7. Serve warm, optionally with a scoop of vanilla ice cream or a dollop of yogurt.

Nutrient Information (per serving, without ice cream or yogurt):

- Calories: Approximately 200-250
- Protein: 2-3 grams
- Fat: 8-10 grams
- Carbohydrates: 30-35 grams
- Fiber: 3-4 grams

Fresh Fruit Salad with Coconut Yogurt and Honey

- Serving Size: 1 serving
- Prep Time: 10 minutes

Ingredients:

- 1 cup mixed fresh fruit (e.g., berries, melon, citrus)
- 1/2 cup unsweetened coconut yogurt

- 1 tablespoon honey

Instructions:

1. Mix mixed fresh fruit with unsweetened coconut yogurt.
2. Drizzle honey over the fruit salad and yogurt.
3. Serve as a refreshing dessert.

Nutrient Information (per serving):

- Calories: Approximately 150-200
- Protein: 2-3 grams
- Fat: 6-8 grams
- Carbohydrates: 30-35 grams
- Fiber: 3-4 grams

Dark Chocolate Avocado Mousse

- **Serving Size:** 1 serving
- **Prep Time:** 15 minutes

Ingredients:

- 1 ripe avocado
- 2 tablespoons dark cocoa powder
- 1 tablespoon honey or maple syrup
- 1/2 teaspoon vanilla extract
- A pinch of salt
- Fresh berries for garnish (optional)

Instructions:

1. In a blender or food processor, combine the ripe avocado, dark cocoa powder, honey or maple syrup, vanilla extract, and a pinch of salt.
2. Blend the mixture until it becomes creamy and smooth.
3. Transfer to a serving dish and garnish with fresh berries if desired.

Nutrient Information (per serving):

- Calories: Approximately 200-250
- Protein: 3-4 grams
- Fat: 12-15 grams
- Carbohydrates: 25-30 grams
- Fiber: 6-8 grams

Baked Apples with Cinnamon and Sugar

- Serving Size: 1 serving
- Prep Time: 30 minutes

Ingredients:

- 1 apple
- 1 tablespoon brown sugar
- 1/2 teaspoon cinnamon
- 1/4 cup rolled oats
- 1 tablespoon of finely chopped nuts such as almonds and walnuts
- 1/2 tablespoon butter (optional)

- Greek yogurt for topping (optional)

Instructions:

1. Preheat the oven to 375°F (190°C).
2. Core the apple and scoop out a bit of the center to create a cavity.
3. In a bowl, mix brown sugar, cinnamon, rolled oats, chopped nuts, and butter if using.
4. Fill the apple cavity with the oat mixture.
5. Place the apple on a baking sheet and bake for about 20-25 minutes or until it's soft and the topping is golden.
6. If desired, top with a dollop of Greek yogurt and serve.

Nutrient Information (per serving, without optional ingredients):

- Calories: Approximately 200-250
- Protein: 3-4 grams
- Fat: 5-7 grams
- Carbohydrates: 40-45 grams
- Fiber: 6-8 grams

- Serving Size: 2 cookies
- Prep Time: 30 minutes

Ingredients:

- 1/2 cup rolled oats
- 1/4 cup whole-wheat flour
- 1/4 cup chopped nuts, such as almonds and walnuts
- 1/4 cup raisins
- 1/4 cup honey or maple syrup
- 1/4 cup applesauce
- 1/2 teaspoon vanilla extract
- 1/4 teaspoon cinnamon
- A pinch of salt

Instructions:

1. Preheat the oven to 350°F (175°C).
2. In a bowl, mix rolled oats, whole-wheat flour, chopped nuts, raisins, honey or maple syrup, applesauce, vanilla extract, cinnamon, and a pinch of salt.
3. Drop spoonfuls of the cookie dough onto a baking sheet.
4. Bake for about 12-15 minutes or until the cookies are golden brown.

Nutrient Information (per 2 cookies):

- Calories: Approximately 150-200
- Protein: 3-4 grams
- Fat: 5-7 grams
- Carbohydrates: 25-30 grams
- Fiber: 2-3 grams

- **Serving Size:** 1 serving
- **Prep Time:** 10 minutes

Ingredients:

- 1 cup of mixed berries (frozen), such as blueberries, raspberries, and strawberries
- 1/4 cup fresh mint leaves
- 1/2 lime, juiced
- 1 tablespoon of maple syrup or honey, if preferred
- Fresh mint sprig for garnish (optional)

Instructions:

1. In a blender, combine the frozen mixed berries, fresh mint leaves, lime juice, and honey or maple syrup (if using).
2. Blend until smooth and creamy.
3. Transfer the sorbet to a serving dish and garnish with a fresh mint sprig.
4. Serve immediately for a refreshing and healthy dessert.

Nutrient Information (per serving, without optional ingredients):

- Calories: Approximately 100-150
- Protein: 1-2 grams
- Fat: 0-1 gram
- Carbohydrates: 25-30 grams
- Fiber: 4-5 grams

- **Serving Size:** 1 serving
- **Prep Time:** 20 minutes

Ingredients:

- 1 ripe banana
- 1/2 teaspoon cinnamon
- 1 tablespoon chopped almonds
- Optional for drizzling: maple syrup or honey

Instructions:

1. Preheat the oven to 375°F (190°C).
2. Leave the banana peel on and place the whole banana on a baking sheet.
3. Sprinkle cinnamon over the banana and bake for about 15-20 minutes or until the banana is soft and the skin is browned.
4. Remove the banana from the oven and let it cool slightly.
5. Cut the banana open, and top it with chopped almonds and a drizzle of honey or maple syrup if desired.
6. Serve for a naturally sweet and satisfying dessert.

Nutrient Information (per serving, without optional ingredients):

- Calories: Approximately 100-150
- Protein: 2-3 grams
- Fat: 3-4 grams
- Carbohydrates: 20-25 grams
- Fiber: 3-4 grams

CONCLUSION/BONUS

As we draw the curtains on 'The American Blue Zones Cookbook, we arrive at the culmination of a journey—a journey that transcends mere recipes and ingredients, and delves deep into the essence of a vibrant, nourished life.

In these pages, we've explored not just the flavors of diverse cultures but also the wisdom of societies known for their longevity. We've uncovered the significance of the Blue Zones diet and its transformative potential, providing you with a compass to navigate your own path to wellness.

But this conclusion is not an endpoint; rather, it marks the beginning of a new chapter in your journey. It's a call to action—a call to embrace the lessons learned, the flavors savored, and the connections made through food. It's an invitation to infuse your daily meals with the vitality and balance that the Blue Zones offer.

May this book linger in your kitchen, guiding your choices and inspiring your culinary adventures. Let it remind you that each meal is an opportunity for nourishment, each ingredient a tribute to health, and each recipe a celebration of life itself.

As you savor the last chapter of this culinary saga, remember: the journey to longevity and well-being is not just about what's on your plate, but the joy, connection, and wisdom that you bring to every meal. Here's to a life filled with flavorful nourishment, shared moments, and the enduring wisdom of the Blue Zones. Cheers to a journey well begun!

BONUS

As an expression of our gratitude, we offer you a special bonus gift. Scan the QR code to access our meal planner, weight management tracker, and blood sugar monitoring tools. These resources are designed to provide ongoing support as you pursue better health.

If you have derived value from this cookbook and found it beneficial, **we kindly request you to write a review for us on Amazon.** Your review will guide us in developing top-quality resources for people who are committed to their health. Your input and review are immensely important to us, and we express our gratitude in advance for your time and insights.

Thank you for embarking on this journey with us. We extend our best wishes for your continued success in your pursuit of health and wellness.